JUL   2011

Praise for *When Sex Hurts*

"Finally, an up to date, comprehensive source of information for women suffering from sexual pain. I will recommend this book to my patients."

> —Yitzchak Binik, Professor of Psychology, McGill University, Director, Sex and Couple Therapy Service, McGill University Health Center

"*When Sex Hurts* should be on the shelf of every gynecologist and nurse practitioner for women's health. This volume is the consummate reference for a serious problem too often minimized by clinicians because of their lack of knowledge."

> —Alan M. Altman, MD, President, International Society for the Study of Women's Sexual Health (ISSWSH), author of *Making Love the Way We Used to . . . or Better*

D0873573

when
sex
hurts

when
sex
hurts

A WOMAN'S GUIDE
TO BANISHING SEXUAL PAIN

Andrew Goldstein, MD
Caroline Pukall, PhD
and Irwin Goldstein, MD

Da Capo
LIFE
LONG

A Member of the Perseus Books Group

Copyright © 2011 by Andrew Goldstein, MD, and Caroline Pukall, PhD
Illustrations by Marie Dauenheimer, MA, CMI

Designed by Trish Wilkinson
Set in 11.5 point Goudy Old Style

Library of Congress Cataloging-in-Publication Data

Goldstein, Andrew, M.D.
    When sex hurts : a woman's guide to banishing sexual pain / Andrew Goldstein and Caroline Pukall.
        p.   cm.
    Includes bibliographical references and index.
    ISBN 978-0-7382-1398-9 (alk. paper)
    1. Dyspareunia—Popular works. 2. Women—Diseases—Popular works.
I. Pukall, Caroline F. II. Title.
RC560.D97G65 2011
616.85'83—dc22   2010036697

First Da Capo Press edition 2011
ISBN: 978-0-7382-1398-9

Published by Da Capo Press
A Member of the Perseus Books Group
www.dacapopress.com

Note: The information in this book is true and complete to the best of our knowledge. This book is intended only as an informative guide for those wishing to know more about health issues. In no way is this book intended to replace, countermand, or conflict with the advice given to you by your own physician. The ultimate decision concerning care should be made between you and your doctor. We strongly recommend you follow his or her advice. Information in this book is general and is offered with no guarantees on the part of the authors or Da Capo Press. The authors and publisher disclaim all liability in connection with the use of this book. The names and identifying details of people associated with events described in this book have been changed. Any similarity to actual persons is coincidental.

Da Capo Press books are available at special discounts for bulk purchases in the U.S. by corporations, institutions, and other organizations. For more information, please contact the Special Markets Department at the Perseus Books Group, 2300 Chestnut Street, Suite 200, Philadelphia, PA, 19103, or call (800) 810-4145, ext. 5000, or e-mail special.markets @perseusbooks.com.

10 9 8 7 6 5 4 3 2 1

Contents

PART III

WHEN THE PAIN IS GONE

Foreword

If you're reading this book, chances are that your story is very similar to mine and those of the courageous women who, in the pages ahead, share just a little of what they've experienced in their quest to obtain an accurate diagnosis of, and effective treatment for, painful sex. After six months of repeated medical visits for the unbearable burning pain I suffered with sex, I was told that I likely had vulvodynia, but that there weren't any medical specialists or treatments that could help me. Countless other women have been told that their genitals look perfectly normal and there's no reason for their pain—that it's all in their heads. If this sounds familiar to you, you're not alone. In fact, tens of millions of women suffer from conditions that cause painful sex, and they are left without answers or hope after multiple doctor visits. Alternately, you may be one of thousands, even millions, who haven't made it to the doctor's office yet because you find it extremely difficult to discuss this very personal and private pain with anyone, including your doctor. Regardless of where you are on your journey to find help and hope, the information and guidance in this book will steer you in the right direction and help you to avoid years of misdiagnosis and ineffective treatment that thousands of women, including me, have unnecessarily endured.

In the pages ahead, you'll hear directly from three highly dedicated and respected leaders in the field of female sexual medicine, who have a combined experience of over thirty years. Their message that pain with sex is never okay and that you don't have to just grin and bear it will ring loud and clear. Furthermore, with perseverance and a holistic treatment approach, your pain can improve, and your relationships can thrive. Don't give up! In addition to teaching you about the most common causes of painful sex, the authors provide valuable advice on how you can advocate for yourself and obtain the best medical care possible—advice they give their own family members and friends when they are confronting a medical concern. The bottom line is that you have the right to be heard and have your health concerns taken seriously! Keep searching until you find a health-care provider who will listen to you and work with you as part of a team.

There couldn't be a better time for the release of this book. As women increasingly acknowledge the importance and necessity of making our own health care a priority, we're looking for reliable information from reputable health-care professionals, which is what you'll find here. It's time to end the stigma, shame, isolation, and embarrassment that many of us feel about this area of our bodies by seeking help and discussing our concerns openly. My story with painful sex had a happy ending, and so can yours! As the saying goes, "Knowing is half the battle." Your journey to healing and wholeness starts with informing yourself, so don't waste any time in beginning. Start today—for a better life for yourself and those who love you.

Christin Veasley
Associate Executive Director
National Vulvodynia Association

Acknowledgments

ANDREW

This book would not possible without the almost limitless encouragement of patients, friends, and family. In particular I wish to thank our agent, Lauren Abramo, at Dystel and Goderich Literary Management for her terrific guidance, advice, and support; Debra Gordon for her invaluable assistance in molding and shaping this book; our editor, Renee Sedliar, for her enthusiasm about this subject and the women who suffer with sexual pain; Ruth Bradford, Laurilee Roybal, and Hilliary Tolson for their extraordinary professionalism, empathy, and commitment. It is invaluable both to me and to our patients.

I give a huge thank you and I love you to Gail. I couldn't even contemplate writing this book without your constant encouragement, support, and love. Mimi, Julia, and Lena, you are the lights of my life. I thank my entire family for their enthusiastic support of all of my projects.

Caroline and Irwin, your caring, compassion, attention to detail, and incredible hard work never cease to amaze me. I surely couldn't have done this book without you.

I also thank my colleagues who have taught me so much: Lara Burrows, Marianne Brandon, Susan Kellogg, Stanley Marinoff, Kurt Christopher, Amy Stein, Jennifer Chu, Pam Morrison, Gordon Davis, Lynnette Margeson, Hope Haefner, Libby Edwards, Michael Krychman, Sheryl Kingsberg, and many more.

CAROLINE

I would like to thank my mentor, Irv Binik, for all of his support throughout the years and for teaching me how to see the bigger picture. A heartfelt thank you goes to Andrew Goldstein and Irwin Goldstein for their total dedication to helping their patients and their belief in me as a cowriter of this book; I would not have done this without you! Many thanks to our agent, Lauren Abramo, for her wonderful support and invaluable input; Debra Gordon for her amazing help in transforming this book; and editor Renee Sedliar for her passion and interest in the topic of vulvar pain. I must also express endless gratitude to my colleagues for keeping female sexuality at the forefront of scientific consciousness and to my graduate students, past and present, for their eagerness and determination to understand sexual pain through our meaningful research. I cannot express enough appreciation to my husband, Michael, for his unending support and love and to my twins, Jakob and Ahnya, for giving their mom a totally unique perspective on life and lots of reasons to laugh.

IRWIN

I want to thank Caroline and Andrew for their commitment to women's sexual health, first brought to my attention through their attendance at the International Society for the Study of Women's Sexual Health (ISSWSH). You have both served on that board with me tirelessly, and now we all serve as editors of *The Journal of Sexual Medicine* (JSM). It has been a source of pride to work with you on these projects for sexual medicine professionals. Writing this book has been an opportunity for us to work together once again, this time with the goal of helping women everywhere— thank you! And to the woman who means the most to me, who labors beside me helping our patients, putting together the JSM, serving ISSWSH, raising our children, babysitting our grand-children, and inspiring me every day, thank you, Sue.

🎗 Introduction

Why a book about sexual pain? Because sexual pain, or dyspareunia, as the medical profession calls it, is a growing epidemic affecting women throughout the world, and few doctors know how to diagnose or treat it! That means women like you get bounced from doctor to doctor and spend years in unnecessary agony as their lives spiral out of control. By the time women like you find us, they are exhausted, hopeless, and furious: furious at doctors who refuse to take them seriously; at husbands, boyfriends, and partners who refuse to accept the reality of their pain; and at themselves for what they perceive as a weakness within.

We wrote this book because as two physicians (Andrew and Irwin) and a psychologist (Caroline) specializing in sexual pain, we can only help so many women ourselves. A couple of years ago, we coedited the first textbook on sexual pain to educate physicians; now, we want to educate you, the patient, so you can learn about your condition and take an active role in its management.

Before you dive into the book, however, let us tell you a bit about ourselves and the book itself.

ANDREW SPEAKS

After residency, I fully expected to become the typical ob-gyn, delivering babies and performing pap smears and surgeries. Yet, when I entered practice, I was surprised by the number of women who confided in me about problems with their sex lives. Initially, I focused my energy and research on the many women who complained of decreased libido. However, after it became known among my colleagues at Johns Hopkins Hospital that I had an interest in sexual medicine, I was soon overwhelmed by the many desperate women who had pain when they had—or tried to have—sex. And my career path changed.

I grew to recognize the "pain" patients before I even talked to them—for while the low-libido women came in unhappy, the pain patients came in despondent. To them, this pain was the most destructive thing in their lives.

I wondered why these women had not found the help they needed. Then I realized it was because the doctors they saw didn't have the training required to diagnose and treat the underlying causes of their sexual pain. Even I didn't have the training. I had attended a well-respected medical school and spent more than 20,000 hours completing one of the top ob-gyn residencies in the country. Yet, I had received just one forty-five-minute lecture on female sexual problems including dyspareunia—and I had finished my residency barely three years before!

I set out to learn everything I could about dyspareunia. I was lucky enough to have several mentors in the field, including Drs. Stan Marinoff, Gordon Davis, and Irwin Goldstein, and to be married to a dermatologist who taught me everything she knew about dermatological causes of dyspareunia (more on these in Chapter 10). For the past decade, I have focused my entire practice on the diagnosis and management of dyspareunia and to conducting research into its causes and treatment.

Over the years, I've learned that it's so difficult to diagnose the cause of dyspareunia for another reason: Most causes are invisible to the naked eye. If you were able to look at your vaginal area, you might see some redness, but in most situations there's no visible wound, no cyst with pus spilling out of it, no ulcers or tears. There's just nothing obvious to explain the pain. And despite major advances in our understanding of pain, most doctors, as you'll learn in Chapter 3, still adhere to the belief that if there is no visible cause for the pain, then there can't be pain, particularly chronic pain. Faced with a woman who says she is in excruciating pain during sex, but unable to see any obvious reason for it, they give up.

Often they send their patients to psychiatrists, psychologists, and sex therapists to solve the problem. While therapy is definitely a critical component of any treatment for sexual pain (after all, Caroline is a clinical psychologist!), the underlying medical problem must also be addressed. A good analogy is depression; while therapy and medication each work well to resolve depression, the two work best together.

As you'll see throughout the book, we strongly support a multifaceted approach to treatment, one encompassing medical, psychological, and physical therapies, which, by necessity, involves a team of professionals, not just a single doctor.

CAROLINE SPEAKS

I also came to this field in a roundabout way. I knew early on in my psychology studies that sexuality was my area of interest, but I was unsure as to what specific sexuality area to study; at the same time, I was taking many pain courses and was interested in the brain and how it processes pain. While finishing my undergraduate degree at McGill University in Canada, I volunteered as a research assistant at the Laboratory for the Biopsychosocial Study of Sexuality, where I was involved in several different studies. I worked in the area of orgasm research among other topics, but what really sparked my interest was a treatment outcome study for women with dyspareunia. I was fortunate to work with Sophie Bergeron and Irv Binik on this study (more on this study in Chapter 14). It was my job to explain the study to the women and record pain ratings during gynecological examinations. It never ceased to amaze me how healthy their genitals could appear and yet how much agony the slightest touch of a cotton swab triggered.

I was also struck by how much the pain disrupted their lives and how much distress it caused. That's when I knew I had found my area of specialty—proving that the pain from which these women suffered was not purely psychological and giving something useful back to them. My interest in this area, combined with my extensive knowledge of pain and how to assess it, led me to think about ways in which to study dyspareunia in order to validate these women's experiences.

My research showed that the pain was indeed in the genitals and not "in the head," or imagined. I also found that women with vestibulodynia showed many characteristics (hypersensitivity in other body areas, higher pain-unpleasantness ratings, brain-activation patterns, to name a few) typical of chronic pain patients, further strengthening my belief that the pain was real. This pain condition seemed to act like other pain conditions; perhaps the fact that it affected sex to such an extent threw many health professionals so off kilter that they could not see it as a pain problem.

I have since focused my career on examining vestibulodynia in many different ways. I have an active research laboratory filled with dedicated students who are working on many projects, including developing treatments for vulvodynia, researching intimate relationships of women with vulvodynia, and other exciting topics. I also do my best to present my work at many conferences in order to educate health professionals about this condition and to dispel the myth that women with dyspareunia are imagining the pain. It is my goal to share knowledge with others and to help women with this condition as much as possible. That is why Andrew, Irwin, and I are writing this book!

IRWIN SPEAKS

I began practicing sexual medicine in 1976 under the guidance of Robert J. Krane, focusing at the time on treating men with erectile dysfunction. With the advent of pills to treat men's erectile problems, my office phone started ringing. It was women seeking help, demanding help, desperate for help for their sexual problems. I referred them to our university gynecologists, who asked that I treat these women instead. At the time they had neither the training nor the understanding to be able to help, whereas I was already treating men for their sexual health problems. I recognized the need of both sexes for care and soon realized I was no longer a urologist but a sexual medicine physician.

Over the years I have cared for women with problems of sexual desire, arousal, orgasm, and/or pain, but by far the most devastating is that of sexual pain. I have been hearing Caroline present at the International Society for the Study of Women's Sexual Health (ISSWSH) for years on her concepts of sexual pain in women. After I met Andrew at ISSWSH, we had the opportunity to share our concepts about what causes sexual pain disorders and the optimal treatments for the various problems. While Andrew had vast surgical experience, I was armed with the basic science knowledge of the hormonal dependence of the genital tissue, based on work by Abdulmaged Traish and Noel Kim in our basic science laboratory, with research funded for over twenty years by the National Institutes of Health.

Today my practice is richer for having met both Caroline and Andrew earlier in my career. We share a passion for sexual medicine, Caroline and I share an alma mater, and Andrew and I share a name, although we are not related. Today I take joy in the many women whom we have helped through their pain to a more comfortable life.

ABOUT THE BOOK

When Sex Hurts is divided into three sections. The first section outlines the problem, explains the vaginal/vulvar/reproductive anatomy, discusses how to find and work with your health-care team, describes a complete examination and medical workup for dyspareunia, and offers some options to keep your relationship on steady ground while you search for and undergo treatment. It also provides a detailed overview of pain itself: the types of pain, why we feel pain, why it is so challenging to treat.

The second section forms the core of the book. Each chapter provides an in-depth review of one or more causes of dyspareunia, including symptoms, diagnosis, and treatment options.

The final section is devoted to helping you get your life back, including your sexual life, once your pain improves. We also look at where the field is going in terms of research.

A few explanations about the way the book is written: We tried to write for the broadest possible audience, clearly explaining medical terms and procedures to provide you with the knowledge you need in order to understand what your doctor tells you. We also don't want you to be offended that we refer to your partners as male. We know that some of you have female partners; we are just going with the majority.

Finally, because we have written this book together, to avoid awkwardness when we want to say something individually, we put the name of the person speaking—for instance, I (Andrew)—in parentheses when this occurs.

You will see various exercises sprinkled throughout the book. They are an important part of your education, so we encourage you (and your partner) to complete them as directed.

As you make your way through this book and learn more about your own body and your pain, as well as possible underlying causes and treatments, we want you to keep one thing in the front of your mind: You pain is real and, in nearly all cases, very treatable. That's why we wrote *When Sex Hurts*—to provide help, support, and, most of all, relief, to you and the millions of women we know are out there.

So, here are five fundamentals we want you to remember as you read *When Sex Hurts*:

1. Sex should not hurt.
2. Sex should feel good.
3. Sex should occur when and how *you* want it.
4. Sex should be part of a healthy relationship.
5. Sex should not be the centerpiece of a healthy relationship.

As Amy, a woman who has suffered with vulvodynia (a common cause of sexual pain) for most of her thirty-two years, wrote when we asked what she would tell other women, "Don't give up trying to get better, and know that anything is possible."

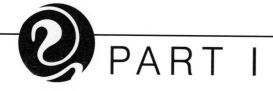

PART I

Essential Background Information

GETTING STARTED ON YOUR ROAD TO RECOVERY

CHAPTER 1

Painful Sex

AN OVERVIEW

> Sex has such an intense impact on how you see yourself and how you relate to other people. It penetrates every relationship. . . . In fact, it is the central issue in any relationship whether the couple is aware of it or not. The nine years of sexual pain I lived through were an emotional hell.
>
> —ANNIE, THIRTY

It's been ten years, but Annie, now thirty, remembers the doctor's words as if it were yesterday. She'd gone to her mother's gynecologist for what she thought was a highly unusual and, truth be told, embarrassing problem: She couldn't have sex. It simply hurt too much. After examining her, the doctor said, "You have a perfectly normal anatomy, but, sweetheart, if you're as tense with your boyfriend as you are with me, it's no wonder it doesn't work."

While those words, and the complete lack of empathy they exhibited, did nothing to help with her problem, they made Annie decide to become a doctor so other women could find someone with more compassion. Many other women like Annie, like you—more than 20 million American women alone—will experience painful sex in their lifetime. You've been bouncing from doctor to doctor and spending thousands of dollars seeking help to no avail. Even if you have found a doctor to correctly diagnose your condition, chances are you haven't found much relief from the recommended treatments. Instead, you've spent years in agony, with pain so severe it feels as if acid is being poured on your skin or a knife inserted into your vagina.

Annie knows the drill well. From the first time she tried to have intercourse, she had lived in a world of pain, doubt, and frustration. The first time her boyfriend tried to enter her, she told us, she screamed in pain. "It felt like he was stabbing me, like I was being torn apart. It was horrifically painful."

The two thought maybe Annie just needed to relax. And she tried. But nothing—not alcohol, not Valium, not even her pleas that he just "rape me"—worked. "I wanted to be normal so bad that I kept asking him to do pretty much anything he wanted," she recalled. "'Just close your eyes and go in there; it doesn't matter if I'm in pain,' I told him. But he was too good a guy to hurt me, and he couldn't do it."

It took another nine years—years filled with dozens of doctor visits, ruined relationships, and the certainty that she was crazy—before Annie found me (Andrew), and I diagnosed her with provoked vestibulodynia (PVD), a condition in which the slightest touch to the vulvar area results in excruciating pain. You will learn more about the causes of PVD in Chapter 6. Suffice it to say, as many as 6 million American women suffer from this syndrome, which may have a dozen or more causes. Nearly 60 percent report visiting three or more health-care providers to obtain a diagnosis, and an astounding 40 percent remain undiagnosed.[1]

In fact, as many as 40 percent of women with sexual pain don't even seek medical care! They think that some level of pain or discomfort during sex is normal. Others are simply too embarrassed to talk to their doctor or don't know how to bring the topic up. If this sounds familiar, take heart—we'll give you the tools to get you the help you need and deserve.

The problem is that painful sex doesn't just occur in the bedroom. It infiltrates every aspect of your life. Many women feel it destroys their very sense of who they are. "I was very shut off physically for three years and am still recovering from that," says Sheila. "I have a hard time being sexual because I don't want to lead my fiancé on into thinking we are going to try to have sex when I am just not ready yet. For me, the pain really affected me more emotionally than it did physically."

The National Vulvodynia Association reports that women like you find the pain of dyspareunia affects far more than your ability to have sex. It affects your ability to function in the everyday world, forcing you to leave careers and to limit physical activities. Some women we've met can't even handle the pain of sitting long enough to drive a car, so they become virtual prisoners in their homes.

"I haven't had sex since I was forty-two," says Patty, now forty-nine. "I cannot wear underwear or pants or anything around my vulva. I wear long skirts with no underwear all year. I bought a special bike seat with a hole in the middle so when I ride nothing rubs against my vulva." Patty used to express her sexuality through salsa dancing. Now that the pain has spread to her entire pelvic floor and hips, it hurts too much to merengue, so the dancing, her last vestige of sensuality after years of sexual pain, is out.

As you can see—and as you may well know—such pain soon becomes the focus of a woman's life. No wonder a study published in 2007 found that 42 percent of women with dyspareunia felt they had no control over their lives and 60 percent felt they had no control over their bodies.[2]

THE LONG JOURNEY FOR HELP

> After the first month, I began to experience slight pain upon sexual intercourse. After three months, sexual intercourse was completely impossible and still is today (two years later). I went to numerous physicians only to hear it was a yeast infection, a bruised pelvic bone, or "just in my head" because I was nervous. I went through much emotional distress, anxiety, and hopelessness. My family and I have spent over $2,500 on doctor bills and laboratory tests. I had everything done on me, including numerous pap smears, pelvic exams, two ultrasounds, an upper GI panel, kidney tests, and a barium enema. Until three months ago, when my doctor finally diagnosed me with vulvodynia, I was hopeless and felt I would never have sexual intercourse again (much less have children).
>
> —SUSAN, THIRTY-TWO

Susan's story is so familiar. The women we see have typically spent years searching for a diagnosis and treatment for their pain. Unfortunately, not only do few doctors know much about human sexuality, but even fewer know anything about sexual pain. For until about fifteen years ago, not only was painful sex not discussed, it wasn't even researched. If a woman couldn't have sex, didn't enjoy sex, or had pain during sex, she was classified as "crazy," sent to a therapist, or handed a bottle of pain pills.

We think this relates, in part, to the way women's sexuality has traditionally been viewed in society—as something to be feared, denied, and destroyed. For instance, in the nineteenth century a woman who masturbated might have her clitoris irradiated, cauterized, or surgically removed. To quell female "hysteria" (i.e., desire for or enjoyment of sex), doctors applied leeches to a woman's vulva and anus. A woman who complained of pain during inter-course (with her husband, of course) was labeled as "frigid." If she could only learn to relax and stop tensing her vaginal muscles, she was told, she could satisfy her husband. Her own satisfaction was not a concern. And why should it be? Women were raised to view sex in terms of submission and degradation[3]; many probably be-lieved that pain was just a natural by-product.

It wasn't until the 1950s and the groundbreaking research con-ducted by Alfred Kinsey that we began to understand and explore the true nature of a woman's sexuality and to view women as sex-ual beings in their own right. Kinsey published *Sexual Behavior in the Human Female* in 1953 to a firestorm of protest, controversy, admiration, disgust, and just plain prurient interest (if you're in-terested, pick up a copy—it's available at a variety of retailers). The interviews he and his colleagues conducted with more than 5,500 women of all ages, races, and socioeconomic levels forever changed the way the world viewed women's sexuality.

Unfortunately, it did very little to change the way doctors viewed it. And even though issues of sexual desire in women get more attention in the medical field these days, sexual pain re-mains misunderstood, underdiagnosed, and mistreated by all but a handful of doctors around the country.

And that's unfortunate, for in the past decade—indeed, within just the past few years—we have made incredible inroads into un-derstanding the medical as well as psychological origins of sexual pain. That, in turn, means we are so much better at diagnosing and treating the underlying causes of the terrible agony so many women experience with sex.

Before we get into the meat of the book—including a list of the conditions that cause dyspareunia—it's time for a brief anatomy lesson.

A BIT OF ANATOMY: FEMALE GENITALIA

When is the last time you really looked at your labia? Your vulva? Your clitoris? Unless you have had a baby and were able to view the birth via a mirror, we're betting the answer is never. That's the reason for this section: to help you get comfortable and familiar with your own body.

In order to understand what's going on "down there," it's important that you know what's what. It is also important that you understand your anatomy so you can be more specific in describing your pain, something we'll talk more about in Chapter 3. Figure 1.1 depicts the various external and internal parts of your genitalia. Let's start on the outside and work our way in.

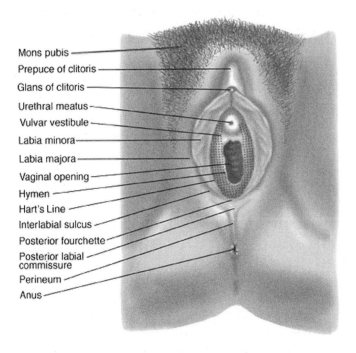

FIGURE 1.1 Female genitalia

External Genitalia

Vulva. The vulva refers to the entire area around the opening of your vagina. This includes the mons pubis, labia majora, interlabial sulcus, labia minora, clitoris and clitoral prepuce (hood), vulvar vestibule, hymen, and perineum.

Mons pubis. This is the part you're likely most familiar with: the pubic mound covered with hair.

Clitoris. The clitoris is the most sexually sensitive part of your body. It straddles the line between internal and external since much of it remains hidden beneath the skin. The part you see is the glans, which is partially covered by a "hood" of skin called the prepuce. This prepuce recedes when you're aroused, as the clitoris, like the penis, fills with blood. You probably know that the clitoris is the site of most orgasms for women. But did you know that the clitoris is basically a female penis? The two organs develop from the same embryologic tissue, so both become engorged with blood when aroused. This type of structure—one that develops from the same original tissue in the male and female—is called a homologue.

Labia majora and minora. Labia means "lips" in Latin, and from a certain angle, the labia do resemble lips around the "mouth" of the vaginal opening, or introitus. These skin folds include the labia majora, the outer folds of skin and fatty tissue that extend from the mons pubis to about an inch above the anus. They are usually covered with pubic hair and, like many other parts of a woman, vary in size, color, and length, depending on the woman.

The labia minora have no fatty tissue, so they are much thinner than the labia majora. They begin at the clitoral hood and extend below the vagina. Their color and appearance also vary, ranging from pink to dark brown, smooth to wrinkled. They contain small oil glands that resemble yellow dots and may also have tiny, raised, pink bumps on the inner surface, all of which is perfectly normal. The area between the labia majora and labia minora, called the interlabial sulcus, is usually quite red, even in women without vulvar pain issues. One other thing to mention about the labia minora: Some women have very small labia minora, and some women don't have any! This is quite normal, as are "uneven," or asymmetrical, labia minora.

Perineum. This refers to the area between the vaginal opening and anus. During labor, this area can rip, which is why doctors sometimes make a cut in the vulva to facilitate birth and avoid tearing. Unfortunately, this cut, called an episiotomy, can cause its own problems with sexual pain (see Chapter 12 for more on this).

Urethra. This is the tube that carries urine from the bladder to outside the body.

Vulvar vestibule. The vestibule extends from Hart's Line (named for the famous nineteenth-century Scottish gynecologist and anatomist Davis Berry Hart) on the inner side of the labia minora to the opening of the hymen. It also includes the urethral meatus, the opening of the urethra, and the hymen.

Opening into the vulvar vestibule are major and minor glands. The major glands are the Bartholin's and Skene's glands. The Bartholin's glands are located in the labia majora and open into the vestibule. If you picture the vestibule as a clock, they open at four and eight. The Skene's glands open on each side of the urethral meatus. Much smaller "minor" glands are found throughout the vestibule. Together, these glands are responsible for about a third of the lubrication produced when you're aroused.

Hart's Line, which your doctor can actually see on the inner labia minora, marks more than just a transition between two body parts; it marks a change in tissue type, an important distinction that will become clearer later in this chapter. This is because embryologically the vestibule is derived from the urinary system and not from the vagina or the outer part of the vulva.

Most disorders involving sexual and vulvar pain are caused by problems originating in the vulvar vestibule.

Hymen. The hymen is a thin mucosal ring that partially covers the vaginal introitus. Despite its relatively minor role in a woman's genitalia and sex life, more has been written about the hymen than any other reproductive structure! And, just to clear up a common myth, lack of an intact hymen is not evidence that one is not a virgin. Even young girls can have a "broken" hymen as the result of exercise or other physical activities. Once the hymen is broken—or "gaping," as it's medically described—its remnants form a perforated ring around the vaginal opening.

Inner Genitalia

Vagina. Vagina comes from the Latin word for "sheath," which makes sense once when you think about it! The first thing to know: You cannot see your vagina. Unless you have an extra speculum hanging around, whatever you might have thought you'd seen down there was not your vagina. That's because your vagina is an internal structure. This tubelike organ stretches from the hymen to the cervix at the opening mouth of the uterus. It is also very close to the bladder, so an infection or inflammation of one organ can cause symptoms in another. That's why you might feel like you have a urinary tract infection when, in fact, you're suffering from vaginitis.

You should also know it's highly unlikely that your pain is coming from your vagina, which has relatively few nerve endings. That's why you can have a terrible yeast infection in your vagina and not know it; only after the infection travels to the vestibule—which is packed with nerve endings—do the pain and itching hit.

Cervix. The cervix is the lower, narrow portion of the uterus. Generally tightly closed, it opens wide during labor to allow the baby to move down the birth canal (vagina). During Pap smears, cells from the cervix are scraped off and screened for precancerous changes.

Ovaries. The ovaries are two small, gray organs, each about the size of a walnut. At birth, a female has more than a million eggs in her ovaries. Obviously, not all are released! However, throughout her life a woman will develop about 8,000 follicles, although only about 300 will reach full maturity and release an egg. The ovaries also produce the sex hormones: estrogen, progesterone, and testosterone.

The ovaries can be a source of pain or discomfort, as many women can attest to after having them palpated (lightly squeezed) during a gynecological exam.

Fallopian tubes. These tubes rise up from either side of the uterus and wrap around the ovaries. Eggs from the ovaries travel down the fallopian tubes to the uterus. If the embryo starts to grow in the tube instead of the uterus, an ectopic pregnancy results, usually causing excruciating pain, severe bleeding, and pregnancy loss.

LABIAPLASTY?

In the past few years, plastic surgeons have begun selling a new procedure: labiaplasty. Believe it or not, this involves cosmetic surgery to the labia to make them smaller and "more beautiful." My wife (a dermatologist and medical ethicist) and I (Andrew) wrote an article about the ethical issues around cosmetic labiaplasty, finding that the procedure is not always marketed or performed with appropriate safeguards. For instance, many surgeons are not properly trained in the procedure, the best way to perform it is unclear, and we don't even know the true complication rate. I know I once treated a woman who'd undergone labiaplasty. The procedure didn't go well, and she had to take an antidepressant for a year for the resulting pain (you'll learn more about the role of antidepressants in controlling pain in Chapter 5).

If you believe that your genitals are so ugly that they must be surgically altered, consider talking to someone who can help you understand why you're feeling this way. Negative feelings about your body can be related to past experiences with partners, shame associated with sexuality, or false beliefs about what genitals should look like. (Hint: Don't buy into the belief that there's such a thing as "ideal" genitals. Female genitalia come in all shapes and sizes. As long as they work well, they are perfect!) Or the feelings can be related to something else entirely. The point here is that you should understand your motivation before you decide to have someone cut into your genitals. Remember: The procedure can result in long-term complications.

CAUSES OF PAINFUL SEX

Each of the conditions listed below will be discussed in more detail in later chapters, but we want you to have a basic understanding of them as you make your way through the rest of the book. Even a brief overview of these conditions will reveal a very important fact about sexual pain: Conditions frequently overlap, and women will often have several underlying causes. That's one reason why you're still suffering.

A reminder: The term *dyspareunia* refers to sexual pain—no matter what the cause. Terms like *vulvodynia*, *vestibulodynia*, and *vaginitis* refer to specific conditions that cause dyspareunia.

Provoked vestibulodynia (PVD). This syndrome used to be called vulvar vestibulodynia syndrome (and, less commonly, vestibular adenitis). But PVD is not a single condition; rather, it constellates at least a dozen different conditions, resulting in pain originating from the entrance to the vagina, the vulvar vestibule. The most common cause of sexual pain in premenopausal women, it is also one of the most difficult for most doctors to diagnose and treat correctly. The most common causes of PVD are hormonal changes, tight pelvic floor muscles, and an increased number of nerve endings in the vestibule. In Chapter 6 we show how you and your doctor can figure out the cause of your PVD.

Hypertonic pelvic floor muscle dysfunction. This condition, also known as vaginismus, occurs when the muscles that surround the vagina, bladder, and anus spasm, causing pain at the vulvar vestibule and leading to pain upon penetration. Tight (hypertonic) pelvic floor muscles can also cause constipation, fissures in your rectum, frequent urination, and problems urinating. In addition, if the muscles are in severe spasm, you may experience generalized vulvar burning, the major symptom of generalized vulvodynia (see below).

Vulvar and vaginal atrophy. One of the most common causes of sexual pain is hormonal changes (decreased estrogen and testosterone) that result in thinning (atrophy) of the vaginal and vulvar tissue. This, in turn, leads to dryness, irritation, tearing, and pain at the vestibule (provoked vestibulodynia). There are many causes of these hormonal changes, including hormonal contraceptives, infertility medications, endometriosis treatments, removal of the ovaries, medication for breast cancer, and menopause. In our experience, hormonal birth control methods (pills, patches, and rings) are the leading cause of atrophy in premenopausal women, thus a leading cause of their sexual pain.

Vulvar and vaginal skin disorders. The skin of the vulva and the mucosa of the vagina are susceptible to inflammatory skin diseases that can cause ulcers, erosions, and scarring. The most common of these disorders are lichen sclerosus and erosive lichen planus.

Interstitial cystitis (IC). IC, also know as painful bladder syndrome, is a condition in which the bladder lining becomes severely inflamed. This causes frequent urination (up to sixty times a day!), severe pelvic pain, and dyspareunia. Of women with IC, 75 percent say that sex makes their pain and need to urinate worse.

Endometriosis and chronic pelvic pain. Endometriosis, a condition in which uterine tissue grows outside the uterus, is one of the most complex and frustrating, yet common, conditions in gynecology. Women with endometriosis often experience severe pain, sometimes only at certain times during their menstrual cycle, sometimes always. In addition to chronic pelvic pain, these women may also suffer from deep dyspareunia.

Generalized vulvodynia. This condition results in pain in the vulvar area even when women aren't trying to have sex. Most often, the pain is caused by a combination of tight pelvic floor muscles and injury to the pudendal nerve.

Gastrointestinal conditions. Conditions such as irritable bowel syndrome and ulcerative colitis can contribute to painful sex.

Infection. Numerous infections, including sexually transmitted infections, yeast infections, trichomoniasis, genital herpes, chlamydia, and gonorrhea, can cause sexual pain. However, while many women (and their doctors) may think an infection is behind their sexual pain, it rarely is.

Pudendal neuralgia. With this condition, the pudendal nerve—which carries sensation from the external genitals, the lower rectum, and the area between the genitals and the rectum (perineum) to the brain—has become damaged or trapped. Women with this condition feel severe burning and aching pain when they try to sit and often have problems with their bladder and bowels.

THE EARLY SEEDS OF YOUR PAIN

Now we're going to take a step back and explore the development of your genitalia in utero by focusing on the embryology of your reproductive system. We think this discussion is very important because one of the most common causes of sexual pain in women is PVD, and one common cause of PVD is related to abnormal fetal development. That's right: The seeds of your pain may have been planted decades before you ever felt the first twinge.

As you know, we all start from two cells: an egg and a sperm. Once they merge and the sperm has fertilized the egg, the resulting zygote begins dividing. Two cells become four, which become eight, which become sixteen, and so on (although not always quite so mathematically neatly). By about day four, you have a ball of about one hundred cells with an inner cavity. At this point, the embryo begins differentiating into the placenta. As the development continues, the fetal cells also begin differentiating into tissues with specific characteristics that will define their role throughout the life span. Each tissue is jammed with various receptors that will provide "docking" stations for the different hormones needed to direct the cells' activities.

In addition, each tissue has its own blood and nerve supply. So, even if you have two tissue types right next to each other—like the vagina and the vestibule—they can have completely different hormone receptors, blood supplies, and nerves.

At about week five post conception, a pair of genital ridges form near what will eventually turn into the kidneys. A week later, the cells of the genital ridge invade what will be the future gonads—ovaries in a female—forming clumps of cells called primitive sex cords. In females, at about the eighth week, primitive tissues called the Müllerian ducts give rise to the internal and external genitalia. These ducts run down the sides of a ridge of tissue called the urogenital ridge, which will eventually become the external genitalia. The ducts eventually develop into the uterus, fallopian tubes, and upper part of the vagina.

Where they come in contact with tissue that will eventually form the back wall of the pelvis, a small swelling emerges, which eventually forms the hymen. Think of the hymen as a kind of fence, a dividing line between the tissue that composes the upper vagina, uterus, cervix, and fallopian tubes and the tissue that composes the vulvar vestibule. The vestibular tissue has more in common cellwise with the bladder and urethra than with the vagina, and it is fed by different blood and nerve supplies. That's one reason why women with vestibular abnormalities often also have urinary tract problems, and vice versa. Both organs developed from the same primitive tissue.

This tissue is not, however, related to the clitoris or labia. That's why women with PVD, which you'll read more about in Chapter 6, can be touched in those areas without pain. But the slightest touch of a cotton swab on their vestibule creates agony. We are coming to recognize that some women have a congenital—meaning from birth—defect that results in an overgrowth of nerve endings in the vestibular tissue. And because the belly button originates from the same tissue, they also have increased nerve endings and sensitivity there. In these women, pressure on the belly button results in pain radiating down toward the vagina.

THE VERY EARLY CAUSES OF VAGINAL DRYNESS

Your vagina is a hotbed of estrogen receptors. That hormone helps maintain healthy vaginal tissue by supporting a healthy blood supply, among other things. So, when estrogen levels drop after menopause, that tissue atrophies, shrinks, and dries up, while lubrication decreases because there is less blood flow to the area. The result? Painful sex. Most doctors just prescribe vaginal estrogen to restore the vagina to health. And that works fine—if atrophic vaginitis is the problem.

But for many women, the real problem occurs when their partner tries to enter them—at the vestibule. Because the vestibule developed separately from the vagina, it also requires quite a lot of testosterone, in addition to estrogen, to remain healthy.

Without both estrogen and testosterone, the vestibule becomes dry and thin, interfering with penetration. The vestibule also has a separate blood supply from the vagina. Thus, because the two tissues—so close yet so far apart—developed from different embryologic structures, treating one has no effect on the other.

(continues)

THE VERY EARLY CAUSES OF VAGINAL DRYNESS

(continued)

This knowledge, however, is relatively new. That's because for years the effect of hormonal changes on the vestibule was hidden. Doctors prescribed estrogen creams for nearly any postmenopausal woman complaining of painful sex. The cream was, well, kind of messy, so it poured out of the vagina, coating the vestibule. Thus, even though it didn't contain testosterone, it helped enough, enabling penetration. But because we're all warier of long-term use of systemic estrogen these days, and the creams cause systemic absorption of estrogen, doctors are more likely to recommend a low-dose estrogen tablet like Vagifem or an estrogen ring like Estring, both of which are inserted into the vagina.

Once or twice a week, I'll (Andrew) see a patient who is postmenopausal and has pain during sex. She'll tell me it can't be from the estrogen loss because her doctor has been given her estrogen. It turns out that her doctor is treating only her vagina. She isn't getting enough estrogen or testosterone to restore the health of her vestibule.

The same problem occurs in women taking birth control pills, as you'll read about in Chapter 6. Today's hormonal contraceptives are designed to reduce testosterone production so that they can be marketed as an acne as well as a pregnancy preventative. Lower levels of testosterone mean more pain in the vestibule.

The treatment I (Irwin) offer these women is fairly simple: They should stop taking the birth control pills and replenish the estrogen and testosterone needed. This can be achieved by applying a special cream containing estrogen and testosterone to the vestibule or using the estrogen cream and adding testosterone systemically with a testosterone gel, pellet, or injection.

EXERCISE 1: EXPLORING YOUR VULVAR AREA

We have come to the first exercise. Now, don't freak out. This is a very personal exercise, one that may make you feel uncomfortable. If that's the case, we suggest that you simply get a mirror and look at your vaginal area until you feel comfortable with it. Then you can try the full exercise with a partner—if you feel comfortable doing it. We don't want you to do anything you don't feel comfortable doing!

For this first exercise, you will need some pillows to lean on comfortably and a large hand mirror. You will also need someone to help you—ideally, this is your partner; if not, make sure it's someone with whom you won't be embarrassed to show your genitals.

1. With no clothing on your lower body, lie with your back propped against some pillows and your legs bent at the knees.
2. Let your knees fall apart, exposing your vulvar area.
3. Pull back any hair covering your pubic area (you can also trim it away, if that's possible).
4. Have your helper hold up a large hand mirror to reflect your vulvar area.
5. If you can, lightly touch each of the external genitalia areas described in this chapter. Have your helper confirm what part you are touching and note on a piece of paper those parts that cause pain. Make sure you share what you learn here with your doctor on your next visit.

BOTTOM LINE

Now that you have the background on the prevalence of your condition, its most common causes, and the anatomy involved, it's time to turn to one of the most important chapters in the book, which focuses on what is likely the most important issue in your life right now: your pain.

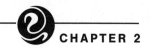

CHAPTER 2

It Really, Really Hurts

UNDERSTANDING THE PHENOMENON OF PAIN

The pain dominates my thoughts all day, every day. I have a hard time working and concentrating because it feels like nothing else matters except this terrible pain. I'm scared that I will lose my job, my friends, and my husband because of this.

—STACY, TWENTY-EIGHT

The pain makes me feel like such a loser. I've had it for six years now, and the psychological aspects seem to be getting worse. I hate going out with my friends or my husband's friends because the pressure to "be normal" kills me. I find myself wanting to stand up and scream that I'm not okay and that I resent everyone that is. And because of where I have pain, you can't just go around telling people. It's not like saying to someone, "Hey, my arm's really killing me today." So I find myself suffering in silence and feeling more and more worthless as the years go by.

—MARIE, FORTY-TWO

Imagine trying to describe the color red to someone who has been blind since birth. What words would you use? How do you make a person with no vision "see" something that has no weight or shape, that is simply a concept in your mind?

That's the dilemma millions of women like you or someone you know face every day as they visit doctor after doctor, desperately seeking a diagnosis and treatment for the terrible pain they feel—pain that has become the center of their world but often has no visible cause.

Before we hone in on the underlying causes and treatment of sexually related pain, however, we thought it would be important to spend some time exploring pain itself and understanding gender-related issues around pain that make women more than twice as likely as men to experience chronic pain.

Above all, remember this: Your pain is real. It is not a figment of your imagination. You are not feeling it because you're angry or depressed (although either could make it worse). You are not crazy! Your pain is the result of biological systems in your body that have run amok. So any doctor, husband, friend, family member, or colleague who tells you that your pain is all in your head (and you should get over it) is wrong. They are invalidating you and your experience.

We will say it again: Your pain is real. You are not crazy.

PAIN DEFINED

There are two main types of pain: acute and chronic. Acute pain occurs as a result of some type of injury to the tissue, whether from an external event (falling and breaking your wrist) or an internal event (an ulcer, childbirth, infection). Doctors understand acute pain; this is what they're trained to treat. They can generally see the cause, find the underlying reason for the pain, and determine what to do. Fix the problem, provide some short-term pain medication, and the pain goes away. Even without treatment, this pain typically disappears when the tissue heals.

Only sometimes it doesn't.

Chronic pain continues after the initial injury has healed. As its name implies, chronic pain can last for months, even years, as many of our patients can attest. The pain you are dealing with is obviously chronic in nature.

There are two main types of chronic pain: nociceptive and neuropathic. It's important that you understand the difference between the two because each manifests and is treated differently.

Nociceptive pain begins in the nerve endings at the site of injury, which trigger the transmission of pain signals to the brain. These nerve endings are called nociceptors. The pain may be *somatic*, originating in the external organs, such as the skin of the vulva, or *visceral*, occurring in the internal organs, such as the uterus and stomach. The pain from endometriosis, irritable bowel syndrome, and possibly interstitial cystitis is visceral; the pain from a poorly healed broken leg is somatic.

Just listen to how Jennifer describes it:

I realized something was wrong with me "down there" when I first tried to insert a tampon at age thirteen and felt a searing, burning pain. There was no getting a tampon in. In fact, I was convinced I had no vaginal entry.

The pain was not much of an issue until I started having sex at age eighteen. The burning/raw pain was unimaginable. Upon entry, I felt a stinging, then as if I were on fire for hours following intercourse. It was so bad, I put ice cubes on my vestibule and into my vagina trying to numb the pain. But nothing helped.

THE PAIN OF ENDOMETRIOSIS: KAREN'S STORY

My life has been totally turned upside down from not only the pain of endometriosis but also the emotional side effects. I started my cycle when I was twelve, and it has never been normal for me. Initially, I got horrible lower back pain. Later, the cramps were so bad I would be out of work for three days, in bed with a heating pad, doubled over with extreme pain.

As time went on, I started experiencing almost daily shooting pains that felt like a knife stabbing though my sides. One day my husband rushed me to the hospital because the pain was so awful. They diagnosed me with polycystic ovarian syndrome and started me on birth control pills. But the pain continued getting worse, including painful bowel movements and intercourse. Eventually, I found another doctor who diagnosed the endometriosis, finding that it covered my bladder, colon, bowel, and uterus.

—KAREN, TWENTY-TWO

Nociceptive pain is likely the culprit behind provoked vestibulodynia (PVD), the most common cause of sexual pain in premenopausal women. Women with PVD describe the pain they feel when they try to make love as a severe burning, cutting, or searing pain, a feeling of "rawness." Numerous studies have found that women with this condition have an overabundance of nociceptors in the vestibular mucosa, the tissue at the opening of the vagina—up to ten times as many as normal! Because women with PVD have so many nociceptors, they feel pain when only a slight amount of pressure is applied to the vestibule. Don't worry; we'll talk more about all this in Chapter 6, which focuses entirely on PVD.

Neuropathic pain also results from an injury or disease process, only in this case it usually involves an injury to or dysfunction of the nervous system, even when it's not clear what caused that injury or dysfunction. The bottom line is that the damaged nerves don't work properly. They send pain signals long after the injury has healed and may even signal pain in a part of the body that's never been hurt.

One example of neuropathic pain is phantom limb syndrome, in which people "feel" pain in a leg or arm that has been amputated. The limb is gone, but the nerves that carried signals to and from that limb remain; they misfire, sending signals of pain to the brain even though there is no discernible cause.

Many of the women we see are suffering from neuropathic pain of the pudendal nerve, the nerve that goes to the vulva. They experience a gnawing, raw, burning, tingling sensation that is not easy to identify, is difficult to locate, and is even hard to describe. It just feels "different" from other types of pain, they say—usually, much, much worse.

Just listen to how our patient Lindsey describes it:

> Everything in my life was going well. I was in graduate school. I was engaged to a great guy. Then I went snow boarding. I fell hard on my rear, and for about a week it really hurt to sit down. That pain went away, but a couple of weeks later I started to have a terrible gnawing pain in my vagina, vulva, and rectum. It feels like a combination of severe burning and rawness. It also feels like there is large, hot ball stuck in my vagina. Whenever I sit down, I can't get comfortable. I had to take a leave of absence from school, and we postponed the wedding until I can be comfortable again. Recently, I had a nerve block and was diagnosed with pudendal neuralgia. At least now I have a diagnosis and am beginning to feel hopeful.

THE INDIVIDUALITY OF PAIN

Because pain—any type of pain—is so subjective, it's difficult to understand and even more complicated to treat, particularly when it's chronic. Even acute pain, like the pain of childbirth, manifests differently in different women. Some women get through the pain of labor with deep breathing and other relaxation techniques; others demand an epidural before they're even undressed. It's the same with headaches. For instance, we know some women who work right through a migraine and others who can do little more than lie in a darkened room for a day or more, waiting for the pain to dissipate.

All of this raises questions like, Is one woman's pain less real than another's? Is one woman stronger than another because she can deal better with her pain?

No. These women simply experience their pain differently. They may even experience different types of pain differently. For instance, maybe you're one of those women who didn't even take Tylenol after her appendectomy, but now you have this pain in your vagina that is so excruciating you can't even sit in the car for more than fifteen minutes. Did your sensitivity to pain change?

No. Every pain and experience of pain is unique. It depends on your circumstances at the time, how long the pain has been going on, and the pain itself.

By the time we see women, the neurologic, muscular, interpersonal, psychological, and muscular components of their pain have become so intertwined that unknotting them is very difficult. That's why it's so important to design a holistic treatment, one that includes medical treatments as well as counseling, massage, and physical therapy. As we treat the underlying cause of the pain and help you better cope with it while it exists, those tightly wound strands will loosen, and the pain will fade.

THE PHYSIOLOGY OF PAIN

Just as food is inextricably linked to the digestive system, pain is inextricably linked to the nervous system, which comprises the

WHY PAIN IS NECESSARY

Although you might wish you could just cut the switch to your brain that triggers pain, doing so would be a bad thing indeed. Pain is there to protect us, to warn us. If you sip a cup of scalding hot coffee and burn your tongue, you stop drinking. If you didn't feel pain, you would keep drinking, burning your tongue, mouth, throat, and esophagus. Without the pain from an infected appendix, you wouldn't go the doctor, the appendix would burst, and you'd die; without the pain from a broken arm, the arm could become infected, and you'd lose it.

There are people who don't feel pain. They have a very rare condition called congenital insensitivity to pain with anhidrosis (CIPA), likely the result of an equally rare mutation in the gene responsible for producing certain proteins related to pain. Unable to feel pain, as babies and young children, people with CIPA shred their lips when they start teething, damage their eyes by poking at them, scald themselves drinking or eating too-hot liquids and food, fracture bones and damage joints—all without being aware of what they're doing. Most don't live beyond their thirties.

brain, spinal cord, and nerves and nociceptors throughout your body. In fact, all sensation is regulated by the nervous system. It's kind of like the fiber-optic network of your body: Nociceptors receive a signal and, using various chemicals called neurotransmitters, pass it from nerve to nerve, by means of an ultra-low-voltage electrical current, until it reaches the spinal cord. There it travels up into the brain, which uses other neurotransmitters to "read" the signals. All this happens in a fraction of a second, of course.

Once the brain reads the signals, it assesses the situation. If it decides you're in danger, it can signal the spinal cord to turn up the volume, or upregulate, the pain signal, making it worse so you get the message that something is really wrong. Conversely, if the brain doesn't perceive the threat as severe, it can send its own signals to the spinal cord to chill out, blocking pain signals from getting through.

How your brain "reads" the message depends, in part, on what else it is doing and how seriously it perceives the threat. That's why techniques like focused breathing, meditation, and hypnosis can be so effective in relieving pain—they "distract" your brain, muting the pain signals. The pain is still there; your brain is just not processing it in the same way. In this instance, you could say that pain is "all in your head" (but not in the derogatory sense of the phrase!).

Pain signals can also be disrupted at the site of the pain itself. That's why running cool water over a burn or having someone rub your shoulders when your neck is kinked reduces the pain sensation. After all, the nerves can only transmit so many sensations at a time. This is important information to keep in mind as you move through the book and we talk about various nonmedical treatments for your pain.

The kind of chronic pain you're feeling—that's a signal stuck in the on position, whether from the nerves to the brain or vice versa. Your brain has learned to feel more pain than the sensation deserves. This process is known as the "windup phenomenon" or "central sensitization." That's why even a light touch with a cotton swab can be excruciating. Our job in this book is to help you retrain the nerves and brain to dial that signal back to low or, ideally, to turn it off altogether unless something really hurts.

WOMEN AND PAIN

In nearly all studies examining gender differences in pain, women are at least twice as likely as men to experience painful conditions

THE BRAINS OF WOMEN WITH VESTIBULODYNIA

I (Caroline) led a study at Queen's University in Ontario, Canada, where I work, that examined the brains of women with PVD, a common cause of dyspareunia. We scanned the women's brains with a magnetic brain scanner, then compared the images with those of a control group (women without PVD). We discovered that women with PVD had more brain cells in several regions of the brain related to pain control and perception, stress, and emotion than women who did not have PVD. An earlier study we'd conducted had shown that these areas of the brain also had higher levels of activation. What isn't clear is whether the pain results in the changes in the brain or if the changes in the brain result in the chronic pain. Stay tuned!

such as migraine, fibromyalgia, arthritis, or back pain. Women with painful conditions also report severer and more frequent pain and have longer-lasting pain in more parts of their body than men.[1] Some of this might be related to the fact that women overall are more likely than men to see a doctor and to list pain as a symptom.

But these gender differences turn up even when researchers compare pain in male and female rodents. Most studies show that female rats and mice have lower pain thresholds than male rodents with, in some instances, longer-lasting pain.

Finally, when researchers conduct experiments to specifically test painful responses in women versus men, they find that women tend to experience greater pain at lower pain thresholds than men and to have less tolerance for painful stimulation, such as temperature pain and electrical shock.

But just as pain itself is subjective, so, too, studies indicate, is the response to pain. Some research finds that the more "manly" men feel, the less they react to pain. It's unclear whether that's related to levels of testosterone or to individuals' own mind-set that "real men" don't feel pain. Other studies find that the gender of the person conducting the study influences how the person being evaluated experiences pain—regardless of the participant's gender. For instance, when a woman conducts the study, men report less pain and can tolerate more pain, particularly if the investigator is attractive.[2] The more attractive the male investigator, however, the more pain women participants report and the less pain they tolerate.[3]

So what's going on?

There are likely many overlapping reasons for gender-related differences in pain perception and tolerance, including genetics and acculturation (the whole "women as the weaker sex" way of thinking).

Anatomy likely also plays a role: Women have more nerve receptors than men, suggesting they may be hardwired to feel more pain.[4] Even something as seemingly minor as the thickness of your skin or the size of your body can affect your perception of pain.[5]

One possible cause of pain-related gender differences is the influence of the reproductive hormones, particularly estrogen, progesterone, and testosterone. For instance, studies find that as estrogen levels drop during the menstrual cycle, pain intensity increases, possibly because there are more naturally occurring "feel-good" chemicals in the brain when estrogen levels are high.[6] You can imagine the evolutionary benefit of this: Estrogen levels are highest during pregnancy and childbirth, thus providing some natural pain relief.

Estrogen and progesterone also affect nerve conduction, as well as the muscles that frequently cause pain. As progesterone rises throughout the second half of the menstrual cycle, the pain threshold drops, and your perception of pain intensity increases. Estrogen has a similar effect, but to a lesser degree.

Meanwhile, other studies suggest that "male" hormones like testosterone (androgens) reduce pain, possibly due to their ability to reduce inflammation, which can trigger pain. For instance, one study found that women with higher levels of testosterone (yes, women have and need testosterone too!) had less work-related neck and shoulder pain than women with low androgen levels.[7] Of course, given that men have ten to twenty times more testosterone than women, this may explain some of the gender-related difference in pain perception we just discussed.

Some experts suggest that the higher rates of pain in women are due to how society thinks of women—as the "weaker" sex more likely to be in distress and admit their pain. We disagree. We see many women who go for years with excruciating pain, assuming it's "normal" to experience some pain in their vulva or vagina.

Listen up, ladies: The pain you feel is not normal! Can you imagine a guy waiting years to see a urologist for pain in his penis?

Women also tend to experience and identify their pain differently from men. While men are more likely to describe their pain in terms of how it feels physically, women are more likely to describe it in terms of how it feels emotionally. This, in turn, results in their experiencing the pain as more severe than men.[8]

This may also be one reason doctors don't take women's pain as seriously as men's (see the next chapter for more on this). That's why it is so important to be a good chronicler of your pain, both verbally and in writing. Don't worry; we'll show you how in Chapter 3.

GENDER AND PAIN MEDICATION

In addition to differences in how women and men experience pain, there are also differences in terms of the effects of pain medication. For instance, women are more likely than men to experience nausea and vomiting when taking opioids (morphine, codeine).[9] They also need greater amounts of pain relief immediately after surgery, while men tend to use more pain relief later in the recovery period.[10] Conversely, some medications can provide greater pain relief in women than men, which may be related to genetic differences between men and women.[11]

BOTTOM LINE

Now that you better understand the underlying nature of your pain, it's time to learn how best to describe it so you can get the professional help you need. In the next chapter, we show you how to communicate just that type of information to your doctor. You'll also learn how to find the best doctor for you, someone who not only diagnoses and treats your pain but also listens to you.

CHAPTER 3

Listen to Me, Doctor!

All the doctors and specialists I saw never seemed to know what was wrong with me. I was not confident in them mostly because I kept having pain each month and they didn't know what to do. They treated me like I was a real nut. I was in such pain—and desperate for relief, and to have a normal sexual relationship with my husband.

—KIMBERLY, FORTY-TWO

By the time most women find us, they have been through an obstacle course of doctors, tests, useless treatments, and, ultimately, disappointment and continued pain. One online study of 428 women with vulvar pain found that close to half had seen four to nine doctors about it. Just four out of ten said they thought their current doctor could manage their pain, and 57 percent said their pain had either gotten worse or hadn't improved since they began treatment. Some of these women had spent as much as $75,000 or more on medical care—and still their pain remained.[1] We find these statistics disheartening. And yet we are continually inspired by the perseverance of the women we see and their insistence on finding a doctor who will listen to them—even if that doctor can't end their pain.

Here's what Courtney, a twenty-seven-year-old with vulvodynia, advises women searching for help:

> Don't give up and don't hesitate to seek a second (or third, or fourth) opinion. My search for help seemed hopeless for the longest time. I was only in pain during sex, so it was tempting to just ignore the problem. But I kept trying to find an answer, and eventually I found Dr. Andrew Goldstein. I believe there's an answer out there for everyone who experiences painful sex, but it's up to you to try and find someone who can help. In my experience, most doctors just want to prescribe pain relievers and send you on your way instead of really trying to figure out what is wrong. It's worth it to keep looking until you find the right doctor.

Courtney is so right. Some doctors just want to write a prescription and get you out of their office. Other physicians want to help but just don't know what to do. Then there are the doctors who believe what they were taught in medical school and residency: Sexual pain is a psychological problem, not a physical problem. In this chapter, we show you how to find the right doctor, how to work with him or her to identify the right diagnosis and treatment, and, most importantly, how to be an equal partner in the doctor-patient relationship.

FINDING THE RIGHT DOCTOR

The first step in finding the right doctor is accepting the fact that you need medical help. Unfortunately, we see too many women who suffer needlessly for years because they're too embarrassed to talk to their doctor about their problem. Annette, who lives in Ireland, suffered for twelve years before she finally saw a doctor in August 2008. "I thought it was all in my head," she wrote to us, "that I was imagining the pain. I got to the point where I could barely get through each day. I was an emotional wreck. I cried in the car while I drove to work and cried on the way home. It was all so much worse because there was no one I could talk to about this."

Remember what we've been saying throughout the book—pain during sex is not okay. You do not just have to live with it. Pain is a sign of dysfunction, of something gone awry in your body. You need to find out what's wrong and start on the road to resolution.

For most women, the initial symptoms of dyspareunia trigger a visit to their primary care doctor or gynecologist. But, as we discussed in the first chapter, few of these doctors know much, if anything, about the causes of sexual pain. Although the ideal health-care professional for treatment would be someone like myself (Andrew), a specialist in treating vulvar diseases and dyspareunia, or Irwin, a specialist in sexual medicine, we know that such specialists are few and far between. So, it's up to you to find a doctor who, although he or she may not know a lot about dyspareunia, is willing to learn and to call upon specialists for advice as needed.

Yet, too often we hear stories like Annette's: "I diagnosed myself after doctor after doctor said it was in my head. Thank goodness I am an intelligent woman and I would not take that answer." You shouldn't take that answer either. The pain is not imaginary; it is real! Any doctor who tries to minimize it by implying that you are crazy, neurotic, or a malingerer is a doctor you should fire.

You should also fire any doctor who treats you like Mary's treated her. "When I was leaving one of my doctor's appointments, standing there in pain ready to cry, the doctor pats me on the back in front of the whole waiting room and says, 'Welcome to a man's world. You have a case of jock itch.' I was so humiliated." If you have a doctor like Mary's, you not only need to get out of that office as quickly as possible, you should consider reporting your doctor to the state medical board. Her doctor breached doctor-patient confidentiality, a serious violation of the Health Care Insurance Portability and Privacy Act, or HIPAA as it's more commonly known, not to mention of professional ethics.

Lisa saw five doctors in one year (four gynecologists and a primary care doctor), all of whom told her there was nothing wrong with her beyond the occasional bacterial infection, and there was no reason she should feel any pain with intercourse. One doctor told her, "Maybe this is just the way you are." Another said that she was having sex too much! "That was funny," she says, "considering that I was rarely able to have intercourse at all!" She finally received a diagnosis of PVD from a dermatologist who specialized in sexual pain.

As you can see from these women's stories, you may need to see several doctors before finding the right one. You can reduce the number by focusing on the right criteria:

Instead of

- the type of insurance your doctor accepts
- how well the office is run
- whether the office conveniently located

focus on the following when choosing a doctor:

- his or her interpersonal skills
- his or her medical skills (and how current the doctor keeps them)

One national poll found that people were much more interested in a doctor's interpersonal skills than his or her medical judgment or experience. The most important attributes, said participants, were doctors who treated their patients with dignity and respect, listened carefully, and were easy to talk to.[2] We agree—up to a point. You still want a doctor who keeps current with the medical literature, reading the major journals in his or her field and attending pertinent medical meetings. Medicine changes so quickly that no doctor should rely on what he or she learned in medical school. Bottom line: You need a doctor who is willing to search for and read current medical literature.

You should also remain open as to what type of doctor you see. The specialists most likely to be able to help you are not just gynecologists and sexual medicine physicians but urologists, dermatologists,

WHO CAN HELP?

The following organizations offer advice and support, and most also provide the names of health-care professionals in your area who have experience with dyspareunia and the underlying conditions that cause it.

The International Society for the Study of Vulvovaginal
  Disorders (ISSVD)
    www.issvd.org

The National Vulvodynia Association (NVA)
    www.nva.org

The International Society for the Study of Women's Sexual
  Health (ISSWSH)
    www.isswsh.org

The Section on Women's Health of the American Physical
  Therapy Association (APTA)
    www.womenshealthapta.org

Interstitial Cystitis Association (ICA)
    www.ichelp.org

Institute for Sexual Medicine
    http://sexualmed.org

internists, family practitioners, pain specialists, neurologists, and psychiatrists or psychologists. You may see more than one doctor. You may have a team of doctors. If you are flexible and follow the advice in this chapter, you should find the medical specialist who can help you. While this may take a bit of trial and error to identify the correct provider, your search may be quicker if you contact one of several different medical societies or patient-advocacy groups listed in the box.

TALKING TO YOUR DOCTOR

Once you've got an appointment with a doctor, you may wonder, What's next? How do you communicate the pain and frustration you've been feeling? How do you get past the embarrassment you feel talking about your sex life with a stranger?

We know it's not easy—not for you and not for your doctor. One international study found just 14 percent of patients said their doctors had asked them about their sexual lives in the past three years.[3] When you ask doctors why this is, they say they're embarrassed to bring up sex, they don't feel qualified to respond to problems if there are any, and they don't have time to open up that particular can of worms.[4] While this might improve one day, the reality is that the proverbial ball is in your court when it comes to bringing up this issue.

Unfortunately, surveys also find patients are reluctant to broach the topic of sexual issues with their doctor. In one study, nearly seven out of ten people said they worried doing so would embarrass their doctor, while 71 percent said they thought their doctor wouldn't listen to them or address their concern anyway.[5]

Listen, you are trusting, and paying, your doctor to manage your health problems—all your health problems. You have a right to assessment and treatment for sexual health problems, especially anything involving pain. Pain, as you learned in the previous chapter, is your body's way of warning you that something is wrong. So, if your doctor tries to dismiss your concerns, remind him or her of that!

Here's a step-by-step list of how to prepare for, and what to expect, at your appointment.

1. Tell the receptionist the purpose of your visit when making the appointment. That way he or she can schedule you for the appropriate time slot. Hint: This is not a fifteen-minute appointment. I (Andrew) schedule at least an hour for a new patient appointment, but I know that's not realistic for many doctors. Clarifying the reason for the visit also gives your doctor a heads-up; smart professionals will do a little research on the side before meeting with you.

2. Ask if any blood tests should be done first. I (Irwin) speak with each patient on the phone before they come in to determine if it would be helpful to have their hormone levels available before their appointment.

3. Track your symptoms. In the weeks or days before your appointment, keep a diary of your symptoms. When do they occur? What were you doing when they occurred? How long did the pain last? What did the pain feel like? The issues you should think about and be prepared to discuss include the following:
   ▸ Itching. Where, when, and how often do you experience itching? What do you do when you feel the itching?
   ▸ Menstrual cycle. Is your cycle regular or irregular, or are you menopausal?
   ▸ Pain. Provide as many adjectives as possible (see "Words to Describe Pain"). Do you feel it all the time? Does it come and go? When is it worse? Does it hurt when you wear underwear

or pants? When do you feel the pain? Does it hurt only during sex or also afterward? Do you have pain with clitoral stimulation? How long does the pain associated with sex last? Can you use a tampon? Does the pain get worse or better at different times of the month? What makes it better? What makes it worse?

We find it especially useful to have our patients prepare a written chronological history of their pain and previous treatments, which we review with them during their initial appointment.

WORDS TO DESCRIBE PAIN

Pain is such a subjective experience that simply finding the right words to describe it can be a challenge. Here are some words to help you get started: "searing," "burning," "stabbing," "cramping," "itching," "sharp," "cutting," "dull," "aching," "throbbing," "gnawing," "jabbing," "hot," "cold," "pressure," "bloating," "numbing," "shooting," "soreness," "constant," "radiating," and "tightness."

4. List the medications you take, and include *everything*, even vitamins, herbal supplements, and over-the-counter drugs like aspirin, acetaminophen (Tylenol), ibuprofen (Motrin), and the like. Even better, bring your medications with you in a bag so your doctor can see the dosage and the drug or, at the very least, make a list with the dosage, start date, and remaining refills.

5. Bring your partner or a friend with you. He or she may have pertinent information to add to your medical history and symptom description that you haven't considered.

6. Bring paper and pencil to take notes. Many people say they can't remember what their doctor told them. Having your partner there will help; so will note taking.

DURING THE APPOINTMENT

Hopefully your doctor will first meet with you in his or her office or, at the very least, talk to you in the examining room while you're fully dressed. Meeting a physician for the first time as you sit there naked, covered only by a paper gown, can be very embarrassing. So, if the nurse tells you to get undressed before you see the doctor, politely ask to talk to the doctor first, while you're still dressed.

Once your doctor enters the room, he or she will typically ask you why you're there. Be as specific as possible. Instead of "It hurts when I have sex," say, "When my husband tries to enter me I feel a searing pain at the entrance to my vagina." Instead of "I'm having problems with sex," say, "I feel a deep, aching pain in my pelvic region all the time that makes it impossible for me to enjoy intercourse." Get the picture?

We also recommend that you use a pain scale to objectively describe your pain. Your doctor should have one available. A simple way to describe your pain objectively is to rate it on a scale of one to ten, with one being mild discomfort and ten being complete agony, the worst you've ever felt.

Your doctor should then take a complete personal and medical history (particularly if you're a new patient). Ideally, this begins with an open-ended question, such as "Tell me what's going on." That's your green light to share a personal narrative of what you've been through. Don't hold anything back. Start at the beginning when the pain first began and continue up to today. Be honest and specific, but try to remain as calm and objective as possible.

Tell your doctor how many other health-care professionals you've seen, what treatments you've tried, and if anything has worked. It's okay if you cry. It is important that the doctor understand the effect this has on your overall quality of life, your relationship, and your ability to live normally.

When describing the pain, talk about it in sensory rather than affective terms. For instance, tell the doctor that the pain burns instead of saying "it's the worst thing in the world." Other ways to communicate your pain include the following:

- Documenting the characteristics of the pain—when it starts, when it's at its worst, and where it is. This is where the journal we discussed earlier becomes so important.
- Documenting what has and hasn't worked in terms of managing the pain.
- Specifying how the pain affects your ability to function. For instance, you can no longer wear pants, drive, or ride a bike because of the pain. Have you cut back on work, given up on dating or relationships, or changed your exercise habits because of the pain? And even though you may think it's too obvious to mention, share the specifics of how the pain has affected your sex life.
- Sharing what you've learned from this book and elsewhere about your condition. These days, people are more likely to get medical information from the Internet than from their own doctor, so it's quite likely you've already done some research on your own. Share what you've learned with your doctor; if the doctor reacts negatively to this information, you may need to reevaluate whether this is the right physician for you. Remember, you want a doctor with whom you can work as part of a team.

You'll know you're on the right track with your doctor if he or she displays empathy, understanding, and acceptance. If you feel rushed or that your doctor isn't paying attention to you (checking his or her watch or PDA is a good clue), you probably need to keep looking.

After your narrative, your doctor will ask some questions. Again, honesty is crucial, even if the questions concern potentially embarrassing topics, such as your sexual history or drug or alcohol use. Tell the doctor if you smoke, how often you exercise, what type of work you do, and about your family life.

Your doctor may also ask you to fill out some questionnaires. For instance, one from the International Society for the Study of Vulvovaginal Disorders covers your past medical, social, surgical, sexual, and medication history (this questionnaire is available on Andrew's website at www.cvvd.org). Other screening questionnaires can help identify conditions related to sexual pain disorders, such as irritable bowel syndrome, endometriosis, and interstitial cystitis. In addition, there are other questionnaires used to evaluate women's sexual function, such as the Female Sexual Function Index, which are available on Irwin's website (www.sdsm.info). You might want to have a look at these prior to your visit.

COULD MY MEDICATION CAUSE MY PAIN?

More than nine out of ten women take prescription medications. Since such medications can cause or contribute to dyspareunia, it is important that you share with your doctor everything you currently take as well as any medications you were taking when your pain began. For instance, chronic use of antibiotics increases the risk of yeast infections, which can cause sexual pain. Hormonal contraceptives, the second most commonly prescribed medication for premenopausal women, are strongly linked with PVD, the most common cause of sexual pain in this group. Medication for infertility, endometriosis, and acne can also affect hormonal levels, resulting in dyspareunia. Even antidepressants, because of their negative effect on desire and arousal, can contribute to pain by reducing lubrication.

THE PHYSICAL EXAM

Although the thought of someone, even a doctor, touching you "down there" may send chills through your body, you need to undergo a thorough physical examination. This is very important if your doctor is to identify the exact location of the pain and develop a potential diagnosis. Tell your doctor you want to watch the examination with a hand mirror, and ask him or her to name each part being touched. Although you may feel shy, embarrassed, or even uncomfortable at the thought of doing this, it will help you understand the pain—and how to get better.

Also ask your doctor to use a child-sized, or pediatric, speculum to reduce discomfort during the internal exam.

Now, let's focus on the components of the ideal gynecologic examination for anyone with sexual pain.

Visual exam. The physician should start on the outside and work inward, looking for skin changes such as thickening, broken hairs, fissures, ulcers, erosions, redness, and changes in pigment. Many skin changes are difficult to see without magnification, so we always recommend an examination using a microscope called a vulvoscopy. This procedure involves spraying a diluted vinegar solution on the vulva. Yes, it stings, but the vinegar also turns abnormal skin white, enabling us to see certain dermatologic conditions and precancerous changes that are not visible otherwise. We then spray the vulva with water to get rid of the stinging. The whole procedure typically takes only few minutes.

If we identify a skin abnormality, we then perform a skin biopsy. We inject the anesthetic lidocaine (which stings for about seven seconds), then test the skin with a needle to make sure you aren't feeling any pain before taking the skin sample. The area should heal completely within seven to ten days.

Cotton swab test. Here, your doctor lightly touches a moistened cotton swab to different parts of your vulva, looking for any abnormal pain response. The most important area the doctor focuses on is the vulvar vestibule, the area between the labia minora and the hymen. Again, be honest about what you feel as the exam progresses. We discuss the cotton swab test in greater detail in Chapter 6 when we discuss PVD.

Internal examination. During this exam, your doctor will take some specimens from your vagina and cervix to test for various abnormalities, including sexually transmitted infections, fungal or bacterial infections, or other types of vaginal inflammation. When we give lectures to our colleagues about this type of exam, we always encourage them to examine the vaginal discharge under a microscope. This is called a wet smear. Alas, a recent survey of gynecologist showed that only 56 percent even had a microscope in their offices! However, don't panic if this is the case with your doctor. He or she can send the smear to a laboratory.

We also encourage our colleagues to send a vaginal culture to a laboratory to determine what organisms are in the vagina. We tell our lab to call us if there are abnormalities (before they throw out the culture) so that we can decide if we need additional tests to determine the sensitivity of the organism(s) to certain antibiotics or antifungals. Don't be afraid to ask your doctor to do this; tell him or her that you heard about it from a specialist in dyspareunia and are willing to pay for it out of pocket if needed.

Digital (finger) examination of the vagina. The doctor should use one finger, not two as during a typical vaginal examination (again, to reduce any pain or discomfort). In addition, the doctor should be very careful and insert his or her finger without touching the vestibule. This exam is used to feel inside the vagina and to palpate the muscles surrounding it. Any tenderness, weakness, or painful trigger points in these muscles may result from a form of pelvic floor muscle dysfunction related to overly tight muscles, an important and common cause of dyspareunia discussed in more detail in Chapter 13. The doctor should also press on your urethra and the bottom of the bladder. If either of these areas is tender, you may have interstitial cystitis, covered in Chapter 9.

At this time, the doctor should also gently press on the pudendal nerve, which supplies sensation to the vulva, clitoris, vagina, and rectum. Tenderness in this area may be the result of pudendal neuralgia, covered in Chapter 8. Finally, the doctor will insert another finger into your anus while keeping a finger in your vagina. Called a rectovaginal exam, it allows the doctor to feel scar tissue resulting from endometriosis or pelvic inflammatory disease, covered in Chapters 9 and 7, respectively.

TESTS, ANYONE?

We discuss specific tests for specific conditions throughout the rest of this book, but providing an overview is a good idea at this point. In addition to the vulvoscopy, skin biopsy, wet mount, and vaginal cultures described above, your doctor should order blood tests to evaluate your hormonal levels. As you will read in Chapter 6, hormonal abnormalities are common causes of sexual pain. Other tests depend on your doctor's findings during the history and physical taking, but may include

- ultrasounds to evaluate your reproductive organs, pelvis, or lower spine
- tests to check for any problems in your abdominal organs, including your stomach and colon, such as a colonoscopy, a barium enema, or a CT scan with contrast

- cystoscopy, in which the doctor inserts a thin instrument with a tiny camera on its end through your urethra into your bladder to check for interstitial cystitis
- perineometry to determine if your pelvic floor muscles are too tight or weak
- electromyelogram, measures the electrical impulses of the levator ani muscles to assess their tone and strength
- quantitative sensory testing or nerve-conduction testing to assess the health of the pudendal nerve
- allergy testing to see if you are allergic to certain chemicals or preservatives
- MRI of the hip or spine to detect structural abnormalities, such as a tear in the hip socket, which can compress the pudendal nerve, resulting in pudendal neuralgia

Most of these tests will be performed after your appointment, usually by other medical personnel.

Also, while the idea of undergoing a battery of tests can feel overwhelming and even scary, we urge you to relax. Remember, we want to find the most likely cause of your pain so we can apply the best possible treatment rather than treating you through a trial-and-error approach.

MOVING INTO TREATMENT

I've visited ten different gynecologists, three urologists, two psychologists, one neurologist, and two rheumatologists. One of the gynecologists is a big personality inside his field in Italy, and he could not find any kind of disease. Other gynecologists, since they could not understand the symptoms, used to tease me, saying that I had pain because my sexual life was "too wild." The urologist told me to see a psychologist, saying my pain was likely connected to certain feelings toward my partner, even though I'd told him the pain remained with all partners. I met with a psychologist for a year and a half, but my mind was completely fine. Even my parents and my boyfriend thought I was going insane and I was just imagining all my problems.

—IRENE, THIRTY-FOUR

Hopefully this chapter has given you the tools you need to become more assertive in seeking the right kind of doctor to provide the right kind of care so that you can avoid the situation Irene encountered. It is likely that you are now at the stage where the doctor is ready to provide a diagnosis and recommend a treatment plan. Part II discusses possible diagnoses and treatments, but we want to remind you that even when you get a diagnosis and treatment plan, your job is not over. You still need to ask questions, be comfortable with the plan, and make sure that you are treated as a partner in the next steps. Below we've listed several questions you should ask about treatments, whether medical or surgical.

QUESTIONS TO ASK ABOUT TREATMENTS

If your health-care professional prescribes medications, ask the following:

- What are the side effects?
- How long should it take until I feel better?
- How will I know if the medication is working?
- What if the medication doesn't work?
- Will this medication interact with any other drugs I'm taking or might take?

- How long do I have to take it for?
- Can I drink alcohol while taking this medication?
- Are there any foods I should avoid?
- Will this medication make me sleepy?
- What if I miss a dose?
- Can I use this medication while trying to get pregnant?
- What should I do if I get pregnant?

If your doctor recommends surgery, ask the following:

- Why do you think surgery is the best option?
- What are the potential complications? What will you do to reduce my risk of complications?
- What if the surgery doesn't work?

If your doctor recommends surgery, he or she may not be the best person to perform it. One way to compare different surgeons is to ask the following questions:

- How many of these procedures do you do in a year?
- How do you define success?
- What is your success rate?
- Have you published your success rates?

It is also important for you to understand that your recovery requires a team approach. There's you and your doctor, of course, but there are other health-care professionals as well, particularly physical therapists and psychologists or other mental health professionals. The therapist is necessary because no matter how well the recommended treatment works to reduce your pain, you still have emotional issues to resolve from the months or, in most cases, years of pain. You also have issues to resolve regarding your views of sex and, most likely, your current and future relationships. The physical therapy is necessary not just as part of the initial treatment program but throughout treatment because the muscles around your vulva and vagina are likely tight, contributing to pain even after the underlying cause has been resolved.

We will talk more about all this throughout the rest of the book. In the meantime, you have one more chapter to go in this first section. Don't skip it! We consider it one of the most important chapters in the book. It will show you how to maintain a relationship with your partner despite your pain.

EXERCISE 2: ROLE PLAYING

In this exercise, you are to role-play with your partner or a friend. The other person should pretend to be the doctor, asking the all important "why are you here" questions. Practice your narrative with this person to make sure you cover all the important events.

CHAPTER 4

Containing the Damage to Your Relationship

> Once the chronic pain began, just wearing underwear, sitting through a movie, or driving a car was enough to trigger excruciating irritation. Of course, intercourse was completely out of the question. For two years, my husband didn't touch me. He didn't kiss me, hug me, or hold my hand. He refused to go for counseling or try other forms of intimacy. Although there were other problems in the relationship, I know that my divorce after just two years of marriage was due in large part to our inability to have sex.
>
> —MARCY, THIRTY-NINE

> How do you tell someone that you can't have sex?
>
> —AMY, TWENTY-EIGHT

As if relationships and marriage weren't complicated enough, add excruciating genital pain and an inability to have or enjoy sex into the mix. It's like pouring gasoline on a fire. The result, as you can imagine, is all too often like the one Marcy experienced—the end of the relationship.

The situation is just as complicated for women looking to begin relationships, as Annie learned: "I remember one man I started dating whom I really, really liked," she told us. "The issue of sex came up pretty quickly, so I told him about my 'problem.' He broke up with me on the spot. Another man with whom I'd had a long-term relationship finally ended it by saying 'it wasn't fair' that he couldn't sleep with me *or* with other women!"

In fact, 61 percent of women with vulvodynia told researchers in one study that their condition affected how close they felt they could be with those they loved, while 44 percent said it made showing affection difficult, and 85 percent said it interfered with their sex lives.[1] In another survey, 40 percent of women said their dyspareunia had led to changes in the sexual part of their relationships, and 21 percent of women said it had increased the stress in their relationships.[2]

The thing is, no matter how much we try to minimize its importance or focus on other aspects of a relationship, sex *is* a crucial part of a healthy partnership. Study after study demonstrates that couples who have a satisfying sexual relationship have happier, stronger marriages. As Amy noted, "Sex had always been a very important part of my life. I had been in a few successful relationships and learned that it was a very important part of the relationship."

Yet, as surveys find, eight out of ten women with vulvodynia and nearly half of all women with interstitial cystitis—two of the most common causes of painful sex—say that the pain "significantly and negatively" affects their sex lives.[3] In one survey, nearly all the women with vulvodynia said they had stopped intercourse at least once because of pain, and more than half (56 percent) had simply stopped having sex altogether.[4] For some women, the pain of sex becomes so overwhelming that they don't even want to masturbate or allow themselves to become aroused, whether or not doing so leads to sex.[5]

Overall, studies find that women with dyspareunia are less likely to initiate sex, are more likely to refuse their partners' sexual advances, and are more likely to have sex even when they really don't want to.[6] None of this can be good for the relationship! You likely have your own story about how your pain has affected your relationship; these statistics show you that you're not alone.

So, if sex is so important to a relationship, and you're unable to have sex, does that mean you have to give up on having a healthy relationship? Absolutely not. In this chapter, we show you how to maintain your relationship as you work through the diagnosis and treatment phases of your dyspareunia so you can, hopefully, emerge on the other side not only pain-free but still with the person you want to be with.

PAIN AND YOUR SELF-ESTEEM

It seems obvious that if it hurts to have sex, you will have it less. Not too much to figure out there, right? Ummm, hold on. You need to understand why you're having less sex. Here's a hint: The actual pain may not be the only reason.

Part of the problem, it turns out, is that the pain you feel has all sorts of effects on your self-esteem and self-image, both of which are strongly linked to arousal. It makes sense: If you feel good about yourself and how you look and feel, you're more likely to become aroused and have sexual desire. Conversely, if you feel lousy about yourself—if you're sick, depressed, sad, angry, and frustrated with and at your body—you're less likely to feel aroused, regardless of pain.[7] Plus, just as pleasurable feelings and thoughts can reduce your perception of pain, painful feelings and thoughts can reduce your perception of pleasure, short-circuiting sexual desire. This is an important point to remember. It means that if you're not feeling any desire at all, the problem might go deeper than the pain itself.

PAIN AND YOUR PARTNER

Which do you think would make your pain worse: a partner who was hostile toward you and your pain during intercourse, appearing anything other than understanding, or a partner who was understanding and solicitous during intercourse, trying to find ways to reduce your pain and make you feel better? The answer is both.[8]

We've known for years that in the general chronic pain category, solicitous, understanding partners provide a kind of permission slip for the person experiencing the pain to give into it. So that person begins focusing more on the pain, reducing his or her activity levels and reporting higher levels of pain.[9] It turns out that the same thing is true with sexual pain. Women who perceive their partners as kind and understanding report more intense pain than women whose partners have more neutral responses.[10]

Why? What's going on? Researchers suggest that kind responses encourage women to avoid sex and reinforce their perception of extreme pain. These responses, the researchers suggest, may also contribute to women having "catastrophic thinking" about their pain (see "Catastrophic Thinking").

If solicitousness makes you perceive your pain as worse, why wouldn't hostility make you perceive it as better? Because when your partner is hostile, as Marcy's partner was, this contributes to greater depression. And depression increases pain and disability among women suffering from vestibulodynia[11] and, most likely, other conditions that cause dyspareunia. Plus, if you're in a hostile relationship, it's unlikely that your partner will try to find ways to be intimate that don't bring on the pain; he may even force himself on you or make you feel so guilty that you have sex with him even though it hurts. All of this can heighten your pain by making you feel more anxious, leading to greater pain.

CATASTROPHIC THINKING

You will hear this phrase used later in the book, but, briefly, catastrophic thinking means perceiving everything as worse than it really is. So, for instance, instead of thinking, "This burning really hurts, but I bet a cool bath might make it feel better," you think, "This burning hurts so much that nothing will ever make the hurt stop," or "I'll never be able to have sex again," or "I'll never be normal again." Hint: If you use the words "never" or "always" when you think about things, chances are you're engaging in some catastrophic thinking.

It's crucial that you try to stop when you find yourself engaging in catastrophic thinking. This is an important part of the cognitive behavioral therapy we discuss in Chapter 14.

We mention all of this because we want you to understand the role that your partner might be playing in your pain. It's also important that you understand the impact of your pain on your partner. It's sad to say, but some men just can't take it. Melanie's husband of thirty-two years moved out five years after her chronic pelvic pain began in 2003. "I'm not sure to what extent my pain influenced his decision to leave," she said, but he was very opposed to her taking narcotics for pain relief.

Lisa, a single woman whose pain also began in 2003, says the worst part of her condition is the toll it takes on her relationships. "You begin to dread intercourse, so your partner feels that you're not interested in him. But you don't want to abstain completely because then you no longer feel connected romantically." She would often force herself to have sex, but when her partner saw how much pain she was in, she says, he felt awful for being its trigger. "You just no longer feel like a normal woman who is capable of being loved," she said.

The men involved with women who have dyspareunia are also very frustrated. Many feel helpless, angry, and depressed.[12] Often, they simply don't understand what's going on. They think their partner is avoiding sex for other reasons, and they take it very personally. They may think their partner doesn't find them attractive and feel rejected. Even men who understand what's going on may inadvertently contribute to relationship problems by avoiding any type of physical intimacy with a woman—even holding hands. Overall, we'd say, about one-third of the relationships we see are in pretty good shape, one-third are spiraling downward but can still be rescued, and one-third are falling apart—often because of other reasons in addition to the pain.

That's probably why we frequently see relationships end even after the dyspareunia has improved. In these situations, the sexual pain becomes a scapegoat for all the other issues in the relationship; once the pain is under control, however, the other issues still remain, and the partnership cannot recover. We'll talk more about this in Chapter 16, but it's important that you not try to pin all your relationship problems on your dyspareunia.

MOVING BEYOND SEX

If you're not having sex because of your pain, how can you maintain a strong relationship with your partner? By understanding that sex is more than just intercourse. It's also cuddling, stroking, and caressing (areas other than the vulva if that's where it hurts). It's oral sex and mutual masturbation (if you can bear to be touched down there). It's what you make it. It's learning what you value in one another beyond sex. It's remaining positive and hopeful that once you find the right doctor and receive the right treatment, you will be able to resume a full sexual relationship. Most of all, it's communicating, communicating, communicating.

One way to figure out if your relationship can survive this is to ask yourself, Does my partner care about me beyond penile-vaginal sex? While sex is a critical component of a healthy relationship, it is just one such component. So, if you can't have sex right now, can you put extra energy into strengthening those other areas: communication, companionship, trust, friendship, and sexual activities that do not lead to pain?

"I have a very loving, patient, and understanding husband of six years," says Lynn, forty-two. "I do not think any other man that has been in my life would have understood like Bruce. I still feel like a woman with him, and I know I am okay!" Bruce makes her feel this way by continuing to treat her as a sexy, beautiful woman. He compliments her on her attire and her body; he touches her often in places that don't lead to pain. He kisses her a lot—for no particular reason—sends her sexy e-mails and texts, and remembers to keep the romance in their relationship, even without penetration.

Katie is also lucky. She's been with the same man since her pain began three years ago. While it's had a major effect on their relationship, she said, the relationship has not only survived but thrived. In fact, when she wrote us, she was planning her wedding. "Although it makes me so sad to think that we will not be able to have sex on our wedding night or during our honeymoon, I think the fact that we have stayed together despite my inability to have sex is a testament to the strength of our relationship."

Rosemary, who at sixty-two is quite a bit older than many of the women we see, has been married for twenty-six years. For much of the marriage, she has been unable to have sex because of scarring from a skin condition called lichen sclerosus. A few years ago, prostate surgery left her husband impotent, but they've worked hard to maintain intimacy in their relationship. "We have to show each other tenderness in other ways," she says. "I would imagine

NATIONAL VULVODYNIA ASSOCIATION

I was diagnosed with vulvodynia during my freshman year in college. Sitting, vaginal penetration and even wearing blue jeans all caused excruciating pain. At the height of the pain, I couldn't even sit long enough to complete a mid-term exam, so I turned it in half-finished and drove straight to my doctor's office.

After being told (misled, actually) that nothing could be done to help me and that no specialists practiced in my state, I began my own quest for help and healing. I did research, located a physician at the university hospital and began volunteering for the newly formed National Vulvodynia Association.

While in college, I became friends with Melvin, who soon became my greatest source of support. Melvin stood by my side, always encouraging me through years of painful days and a seven-year period of trying a laundry list of treatments that provided just minimal relief. Friendship turned to love, and we were married.

Soon thereafter, I finally decided to try surgery for the pain. Two months later, we had intercourse for the first time. A year later, we welcomed our first daughter, Grace, into the world. Since then, I have been virtually pain-free. In 2005, we were blessed with another addition to our family, our daughter Faith. I decided to transform my pain into a higher purpose and eventually became the associate executive director of the National Vulvodynia Association. I feel fortunate to have found an answer for my pain, especially because so many other women do not. It is so important for women to educate themselves and become their own advocates and, most importantly, to never give up hope!

—CHRISTIN VEASLEY, ASSOCIATE DIRECTOR,
NATIONAL VULVODYNIA ASSOCIATION

this is extremely difficult in relationships that are younger and where the male cannot grasp the pain concept."

Well, maybe. We don't think a relationship's ability to transcend physical sex for other forms of intimacy is based on the length of the relationship. Rather, it's based on the commitment of the people in the relationship.

While there are numerous reasons to want a strong relationship, here's one you may not have thought of: It could reduce your pain. At least, that's what Canadian researchers found when they looked at women's marriages in relation to their pain. Women with healthier relationships reported less pain than those whose partners struggled to adjust to the dyspareunia.[13]

So, what can you do to keep that spark alive if you're not having sex? Here are ten suggestions. Keep in mind that these are just the tip of the iceberg; you and your partner should be able to come up with at least another twenty!

1. Give each other regular massages. Set aside at least an hour, and if you have kids, lock your bedroom door. Agree up front that this will not lead to intercourse. That way you don't have to worry and can relax into the moment. And don't worry if, as is expected, you and/or your husband become aroused. We'll get to what he and you can do about that in a minute. Keep this time special. Light several candles, play soothing music, and use scented massage oil.

2. Give each other permission to masturbate. Whether done alone or together, masturbation can help relieve sexual tension, even as it may relieve your guilt about not being able to be sexual with your partner.

3. Bring him to orgasm. This is a corollary to the previous suggestion. You can use your hands or your mouth. Just make it sensual and sexy. We guarantee he will appreciate it!

4. Have him bring you to orgasm. Ditto the above. If it is not too painful, have him use his mouth and hands—gently—to bring you to orgasm.

5. Learn to laugh about it. A sense of humor is critical to maintaining a strong relationship through any challenge, but particularly through a challenge involving physical intimacy.

6. Take up ballroom dancing. We recommend ballroom dancing for several reasons: You get dressed up, so you feel pretty and good about yourself. It requires physical closeness. It is something new that both of you can learn together—and laugh about together (see tip five for more on laughter). Not into ballroom dancing? Find another new hobby the two of you can do together: cook or take wine-appreciation classes together; learn a new language together; create your own two-person book club.

7. Kiss. A lot. With lots of tongue!

8. Hug. A lot. The kind of hugs where you hold each other so tightly you might as well not be wearing clothes.

9. Snuggle. We're talking fire in the fireplace, movie on the big screen, bowl of popcorn on the coffee table, and a warm blanket wrapped around the two of you.

10. Hold hands. All the time. When you take walks. When you go out to dinner. When you go to the movies.

EXERCISE 3: INCREASE YOUR DESIRE

This exercise is designed to help you identify ways to increase your desire for sex. Find a quiet place to sit and think, where you won't be interrupted. Think about your sexual history, about what you have and have not liked. Think about your partner. Now write down at least five things that might increase your desire. Over the next few weeks, try at least three of the items of your list. Does it increase your desire? Does it affect your physical arousal? How did your partner react?

We've seen couples who enjoy making lists of the things they love about each other that have nothing to do with sex. Try this with your partner:

- Write down ten things you love about each other that have nothing to do with sex.
- Keep this list in your purse or in a desk drawer, anywhere that enables you to check it often.
- When either of you becomes totally frustrated with the situation, schedule a "reading of the list."

Now that you have some fundamental information about your pain and what may be causing it, we're going to delve into the medical and psychological causes of dyspareunia, how they are diagnosed and assessed, and how they should be treated.

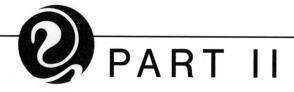

PART II

The Root of the Problem

CAUSES AND TREATMENTS OF SEXUAL PAIN

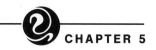
Generalized Vulvodynia
WHEN IT HURTS ALL THE TIME

> I have generalized, throbbing pain while sitting, especially wearing jeans, and sharp pain with penetration. The times when I can handle having sex, I often am bent over with pain afterward, extremely swollen and raw feeling.
>
> —RIANE, TWENTY-NINE

So, you decide this year that you will actually follow through on your New Year's resolution to get in shape and lose weight. You take up running, and to your surprise, you actually like it. Rain or shine, five days a week, you get up at 6 a.m. and run. On weekdays, when the kids have school, you run on the treadmill. On weekends you run on the trail down by the lake.

After about five months, you can run four miles. But for the last few weeks, every time you run, your left leg hurts. You get new running shoes, but they don't help. You stretch more. It doesn't help. You try running on the track at the school because it's softer. Still no better. To make matters worse, you begin to have pain even while walking around.

The guy at the local running shop isn't much help, so you go to your primary care doctor, who prescribes a prescription pain reliever.

That doesn't help much either, so you take matters into your own hands and get a referral to a center that specializes in sports medicine. Now you're getting somewhere!

After explaining your symptoms to the orthopedic surgeon, he puts you on a treadmill and watches you run. Then he conducts a very through exam and orders an MRI. The diagnosis? "It's your knee!" You breathe a sigh of relief: You finally know why your leg hurts, and soon you can start treatment to cure it. Then the doctor tells you that you have a condition called "kneeodynia," which literally means "knee pain without any known cause." The only treatment? Painkillers to improve your symptoms but nothing to improve the root cause.

Now replace the word "knee" with "vulva" and "kneeodynia" becomes "vulvodynia." That's how most doctors diagnose the kind of pain you're experiencing. Vulvodynia itself is defined as "vulvar discomfort, most often described as burning pain, occurring in the absence of relevant visible findings or a specific, clinically identifiable, neurologic disorder."[1] In other words, you're likely to be diagnosed with vulvodynia when your doctor can't find anything else wrong with you, but you still have pain in your vulvar area.

We're here to tell you that most doctors are wrong. We believe that the causes of vulvar pain are, in fact, just as diagnosable as torn cartilage or a pulled muscle. Sometimes the pain is caused by tight pelvic floor muscles, in which case you don't have vulvodynia; you have hypertonic pelvic floor dysfunction. Sometimes the pain occurs because your vulva has thinned as a result of long-term use of hormonal contraceptives or menopause, in which case you don't have vulvodynia; you have atrophic vulvovaginitis, also called atrophic vaginitis. Therefore, the term *vulvodynia* should only be used if there are no obvious causes for the pain. Most of the time, however, a likely cause can be found if your doctor knows where to look and what to look for.

Having said all that, we don't want to completely throw out the term *vulvodynia*. One reason is that as more physicians, media, and politicians become increasingly aware of the term *vulvodynia*, there will be additional resources (grants) to support more research into the specific causes and treatments of vulvar and sexual pain. In addition, if physicians are aware of vulvodynia, they are less likely to tell you that the pain is all in your head and more likely to learn about it so they can treat you appropriately or refer you to someone who can. And, finally, sometimes doctors simply aren't able to find the cause of the pain. Thus, vulvodynia is the appropriate diagnosis until the cause can be identified. So, even though we are not entirely comfortable with using the term *vulvodynia* in all cases, we recognize that it has an important role to play in increasing awareness of vulvar and sexual pain.

Before we go into more detail about the various causes of what we've now agreed to call vulvodynia, we need a bit of a review. Remember the vulva from Chapter 1 (see Figure 5.1)? It's the entire

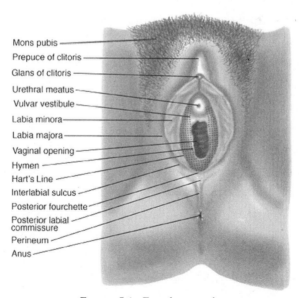

Mons pubis
Prepuce of clitoris
Glans of clitoris
Urethral meatus
Vulvar vestibule
Labia minora
Labia majora
Vaginal opening
Hymen
Hart's Line
Interlabial sulcus
Posterior fourchette
Posterior labial commissure
Perineum
Anus

FIGURE 5.1 Female genitalia

area around the vaginal opening, including the mons pubis, clitoris, and labia majora and minora. Remember the vestibule, or vulvar vestibule? This is the innermost area of the inner lips around the opening to the vagina. Keep these two areas in mind as you read through this chapter and the next.

THE TWO TYPES OF VULVODYNIA

There are two main types of vulvodynia: generalized (throughout the vulvar area) or localized (within the vulvar vestibule only). Either may be provoked (elicited with stimuli such as touch), spontaneous (occurring without any pressure being applied to the area), or a mix of the two. This chapter focuses on generalized vulvodynia (GVD); the next focuses on localized pain in the vestibule, or as we will call it, provoked vestibulodynia (PVD).

GVD, as its name implies, entails a constant burning pain involving much of the vulva and often the vestibule. Marisa, who has suffered with this form of the condition for years, describes it as "like having knives inside of me, a muscle spasm that won't go away." Randi says it feels as if a "lit cigarette lighter" is in her vagina.

The pain can tear a woman's life apart. As Eileen, fifty-two, described it to us, "Vulvodynia is unpredictable and indescribable to anyone who has not experienced it. As a result of the agony the vulvodynia has caused in every part of my life, I am a shadow of the woman I once was or could be." Now, before you freak out at the tone of Eileen's comment, please understand that this poor woman sought help for years, saw more than thirty doctors, and never found any relief because she never saw the right doctor. Based on what you're learning throughout this book, that should not happen to you!

VULVODYNIA: WHAT WE KNOW TODAY

In 2003, a landmark study estimated that at least 14 million women in the United States had experienced chronic vulvar pain during their lives, yet just one-third ever sought help.[2] Hispanic women turned out to be 80 percent more likely to experience this pain than white and African American women. While we can't know exactly how many of these women had true vulvodynia, even if just 20 percent did, that's still nearly 3 million women who suffered needlessly, many without ever seeking medical care.

We're sure that there is no single cause of vulvodynia. The women we see tell us their pain started after having yeast infections, taking antibiotics or birth control pills, or sustaining trauma to their pelvic area. Some can't identify any triggers for their pain; they only know that after years of a pain-free sex life, sex suddenly became excruciating. Others feel the searing pain the first time they try to insert a tampon or have sex.

Today, we understand GVD as creating a form of neuropathic pain, in which women experience an abnormal, unpleasant, painful sensation in response to normally nonpainful stimuli (i.e., the classic cotton swab test), pain in response to just the lightest touch, and much worse pain than should occur in response to stimuli designed to provoke pain.

GVD appears to be a form of complex regional pain syndrome (CRPS), a neurological condition resulting from dysfunctional nerve fibers that overreact to normal stimuli and don't turn "off" when the stimuli end. This process is also referred to as "pain windup," in which the neurons wind up to deliver the pain signals and never wind down.

These overactive nerves feed into the end of the spinal cord, called the dorsal horn. The dorsal horn area acts as a type of gate-keeper, determining which pain impulses get through to the brain and how strongly they are transmitted, as well as when chemicals like endorphins that soothe pain should be released. When the electrical pathways of this gatekeeper malfunction, however, so, too, does your body's pain perception. This is not just in your genital area; we find that women with vulvodynia are also more likely to have other CRPS conditions, such as interstitial cystitis and fibromyalgia.

We don't know for sure what triggers this oversensitivity. In the case of GVD, one of the most accepted theories is that it may be triggered by an injury to the pudendal nerve, a branch of neurons that feeds from the dorsal horn into the pelvic and vulvar areas. This injury doesn't have to be major; in fact, you may not even be aware it occurred. Seemingly minor occurrences like pressure from a bike seat, falling on your butt, or the stretching that occurs during childbirth can injure this nerve. Once the injury occurs, the windup phenomenon can take hold. Our job is to find a way either to calm those overactive nerves or to reboot them like a malfunctioning computer in the hope that they will return to normal.

The thing is, few doctors can diagnose abnormal nerve responses by looking. One reason so many women are told their pain is all in their head is that their doctor can't "see" any problem in their vaginal or vulvar area.

Many women with GVD show significantly increased tone (tightness) in their pelvic floor muscles compared to women without GVD.[3] In addition, treatments designed to improve pelvic floor muscle function (physical therapy, biofeedback, muscle relaxants, and injections of Botox) can significantly reduce generalized and sexual pain.[4] That's why we devote all of Chapter 13 to the treatment of pelvic floor dysfunction.

Trust us: The problem is real, it has an underlying physical cause, and it can be improved.

TREATING GENERALIZED VULVODYNIA

Most women have seen numerous doctors and undergone numerous examinations by the time they finally receive a diagnosis for
their pain. The critical component that leads to a diagnosis of
GVD is an examination of the pelvic floor muscles and the pudendal nerves, which supply pain receptors to the vulva (more on the
role of these nerves in sexual pain in Chapter 8). A knowledge-
able physician can touch the pudendal nerve during an internal
vaginal exam. (In fact, before epidural anesthesia became common during childbirth, generations of obstetricians were taught to
perform pudendal nerve blocks in which they injected anesthetic
into the area adjacent to the nerve.)

Women with GVD typically have both pelvic floor muscle
pain and nerve pain. Figuring out which came first, however, can
be as difficult as figuring out the proverbial chicken-or-egg conun-
drum. That's because if the nerve is injured, it causes the muscles
around it to tighten up. Alternatively, when the muscles are abnormally tight, they constrict the nerves that run through them,
leading to inflammation. It is essential, therefore, to treat both the
tight muscles and the injured nerves to break this vicious cycle.

Once a diagnosis has been made, the search begins for the right
treatment. It's a rare woman with GVD who has not tried a dozen
or more approaches to relieve the pain. Here's a rundown of what
we've found works best, from lifestyle changes to medical procedures and medications, to psychological and physical therapy.

TREATING VULVODYNIA

Unfortunately, most studies on treatments for vulvodynia don't
differentiate between GVD and PVD. In truth, as you'll see in the

next chapter, both types use many of these approaches. While we've tried to provide references wherever possible, our recommendations are also based on our own experiences, culled from work with thousands of women over the years. We cannot overemphasize, however, that all treatments must be individualized. It makes no sense to treat the pelvic floor muscles if they aren't tight or to treat nerves that aren't inflamed. That is why we place so much emphasis on obtaining a correct diagnosis.

Topical Treatments

These treatments work best for women with PVD, but some women with GVD also find relief from anesthetic ointments and creams. They may burn and sting when you first apply them; be patient. The discomfort fades quickly as the area becomes numb. The most common one your doctor may prescribe is lidocaine jelly or ointment. Some women with GVD find that if they apply lidocaine before intercourse, they are able to have sex and even enjoy it! As Alexandra, twenty-seven, told us, "Topical lidocaine on the vulvar area a few minutes before intercourse has been a godsend. I wouldn't have a relatively normal sex life without it. I also use plain Ivory soap to wash and try to keep hydrated because acidic urine also irritates my vulva."

Bear in mind that not all topical anesthetics are created equal. Avoid over-the-counter anesthetics that contain benzocaine, which can be quite irritating. However, emollients such as petroleum jelly and zinc oxide can help. They act as barrier to prevent irritants such as urine from coming in contact with the vulva, while also keeping skin moist and soft.

Other topical treatments that we have found don't work for GVD (but, unfortunately, are still often prescribed) include the following:

- Topical steroids. They are only useful in specific skin conditions such as lichen sclerosus (see Chapter 10) but don't have any role in treating GVD or PVD. Their use can cause changes to the vulvar tissue, including thinning, irritation, redness, and burning.

- Topical antifungals. We see women using over-the-counter antifungal creams such as Monistat (miconazole), Gyne-Lotrimin (clotrimazole), and Terazol (terconazole) to self-treat what they think are fungal infections. And, in fact, women with GVD are prone to such infections. While the medicine can help if you really do have a yeast infection, studies find that what women think is a yeast infection is often related to something else.[5] Plus, over time, these treatments can further irritate the vulva, leading to more pain.

Oral Medications

Antidepressants. Tricyclic antidepressants such as Elavil (amitriptyline), Pamelor (nortriptyline), and Norpramin (desipramine) are often used to treat neuropathic pain conditions like GVD. They appear to work, in part, by increasing levels of the neurotransmitter norepinephrine, short-circuiting the windup pain mechanisms described earlier.

The fact that your doctor prescribed an antidepressant for your pain doesn't mean you're depressed (although many women with dyspareunia are). The dosages used are much too small to do anything for depression. Plus, tricyclic antidepressants are rarely used these days as a first-line treatment for depression. A note of caution, however: Too often doctors prescribe dosages that are too low; so if you have been taking a tricyclic for two weeks or so and have not had any improvement, ask your doctor to consider increasing the dose before you give up on antidepressants.

You should take tricyclic antidepressants about two hours before bedtime. Side effects include dry mouth, tiredness, constipation, weight gain, and irregular heart beats. If the side effects really bother you, tell your doctor. You might be able to try a smaller dose or switch to a different tricyclic.

There is also some evidence that the selective norepinephrine reuptake inhibitors Effexor XR (venlafaxine), Cymbalta (duloxetine), and Pristiq (desvenlafaxine) may help with GVD pain. Cymbalta, in fact, is already approved for use in people with neuropathic pain. Plus, your doctor can prescribe any medication for any medical reason, regardless of what it has been officially approved to treat. Side effects of these medications include nausea, dizziness, sleepiness, and fatigue, but those effects should improve as your body adjusts to the medication.

The most commonly prescribed antidepressants—the selective serotonin reuptake inhibitors, or SSRIs, such as Paxil (paroxetine), Prozac (fluoxetine), Zoloft (sertraline), Celexa (citalopram), and Lexapro (escitalopram)—do not increase levels of norepinephrine. Thus, they don't help much with the pain. They may still be prescribed to minimize anxiety and depression resulting from your pain. However, some of the main side effects of these medications are sexual, including reduced libido and difficulty achieving orgasm.

AN IMPORTANT NOTE ABOUT ANTIDEPRESSANTS

Antidepressants do not work like antibiotics. They require time to build up to effective doses in your body and brain, so give them at least four weeks before deciding they aren't working. Also, do not quit taking them on your own; most antidepressants should be carefully tapered off to avoid a very uncomfortable condition called withdrawal syndrome.

Anticonvulsants. Originally approved for the treatment of epilepsy, anticonvulsants such as Neurontin (gabapentin) and Lyrica (pregabalin) are increasingly being used to treat neuropathic pain like GVD. In one study, 64 percent of women with GVD who took Neurontin reported that their pain improved by at least 80 percent.[6] However, in another study, only 43 percent of women with GVD who took Lyrica had significant improvement in their pain, and almost 25 percent of the women in that study dropped out because of side effects.[7] Side effects of anticonvulsants include sleepiness, dizziness, nausea, and swelling in the hands and feet. As with the antidepressants, it may take several weeks to see a benefit, so be patient.

Injectable Therapies

If you've ever had an epidural, then you've had a nerve block. Nerve blocks are injections of an anesthetic directly into the nerves believed to be responsible for your pain. This is a relatively new treatment approach for vulvodynia. When we were writing

WHAT ABOUT BOTOX?

You know Botox (botulinum toxin A) as the antiwrinkle injection designed to slash ten or more years off your face. In reality, though, Botox, which paralyzes muscles, is used for numerous medical conditions, including cerebral palsy. We're now testing its use for GVD. The drug is injected into a woman's pelvic floor muscles. Several small trials show its use significantly reduces pain in women with vulvodynia. However, Botox is quite expensive, and it's doubtful your insurance will pay for it. Thus, we recommend it only be used in addition to pelvic floor physical therapy (more on that in Chapter 13) in women who have tight pelvic floor muscles that don't improve with physical therapy alone.

this book in early 2010, just one small study had been published on its use and that was in women with PVD. That study, however, found that three concurrent but separate nerve blocks targeting three different areas improved the pain by at least half in more than half of the twenty-seven women participating in the study.[8] If it worked for PVD, we're hopeful it might also work for GVD.

Physical Therapy and Biofeedback

Physical therapy is an important component of any treatment plan for vulvodynia when tight pelvic floor muscles contribute to the pain. We cover this in more detail in Chapter 13.

Lifestyle Options

These options *may* help, but don't obsess over them!

1. Switch to all-cotton underwear washed in hot water only. Yes, that's right—no detergents or fabric softeners. Never fear: The hot water will kill any bacteria and odor.
2. Switch your soap. You want hypoallergenic soaps and creams with no added fragrances. Skip the soap and washcloth for the vulvar area, and just use warm water and a gentle touch.
3. Forget about panty liners. When menstruating, choose dye-free, unscented, cotton menstrual pads or tampons. (Most vulvar specialists agree that the Always brand panty liners are especially irritating.)
4. Choose the right lubricant for sex. We recommend Slippery Stuff or any other lubricant that does not contain propylene glycol, which can irritate the area. You can even use olive oil.
5. Do as the French do after urinating. You may not have a bidet, but you should still get in the habit of washing your vulvar area

with a squirt bottle of warm water after urinating and gently patting the area dry with an all-cotton cloth so you don't irritate it with toilet paper. This also removes all traces of irritating urine.

BOTTOM LINE

We want to close this chapter with some advice from women with GVD. Lisa, thirty-two, when asked what advice she had for other women like her, told us, "Keep going to doctors until you find someone who believes that you have a real problem and that this problem can be treated; don't get discouraged by doctors and friends who don't understand you; join a support group such as those sponsored by the National Vulvodynia Association or the Interstitial Cystitis Association [see the resources listed in Chapter 3]; don't try to have intercourse if it's painful. This is more devastating for the relationship than abstinence. Wait until you get some form of treatment."

And from Janine, thirty-seven: "Don't be mad at yourself or feel guilty for not working hard enough to cure yourself! You must live as well. Don't let the condition be your identity! In this world of bounty, we forget that real problems exist—and this is simply the one we have been allotted. Keep tight to friends and family—they are the real gift."

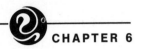

CHAPTER 6

When Every Touch Hurts

PROVOKED VESTIBULODYNIA (VULVAR VESTIBULITIS SYNDROME)

> My first conversation with Dr. Goldstein was a thirty-minute phone conversation. I call it the thirty minutes that changed my life. He listened to my story and asked me a few questions, and then told me he thought I had vulvar vestibulitis syndrome. After confirming it with a thorough examination and office visit that took over an hour, he recommended surgery. Surgery was the greatest thing I ever did. Although the recovery was long and painful, it was nothing compared to the nine years that preceded it. Finally, I could have sex without pain. And it is truly amazing. I just have this feeling that I can't believe I can do this and enjoy it. I still feel like I don't know what I'm doing, but I'm having fun learning!
>
> —ANNIE, THIRTY

Most of you will find this chapter the most helpful because here we discuss the most common cause of sexual pain: provoked vestibulodynia (PVD). One study estimated that PVD affects 16 percent of all women![1] That's huge.

First, an explanation of the lexicon: What we call provoked vestibulodynia your doctor may call just vestibulodynia or vulvar vestibulitis syndrome (VVS). The name of the condition was changed a few years back when experts recognized that only some, not all, cases of vestibulodynia occur with inflammation (the "-itis" suffix of medical words refers to inflammation, while the "-dynia" suffix refers to pain). In fact, we have spent so many years using the term VVS that we find ourselves slipping sometimes; of course, it doesn't help that most of the literature regarding PVD actually uses the term VVS. Regardless, we'll try to stick with the acronym PVD in this chapter and throughout the rest of the book.

Put simply, PVD is pain in the vulvar vestibule that occurs in response to some type of contact. It can be either primary, occurring the first time a woman tries to use a tampon or have intercourse, or secondary, occurring after months or years of a pain-free sex life.

Here's how Annette, thirty-four, who has primary PVD, describes the pain: "Searing, stabbing pain at the entrance to the vagina if penetration of any kind was attempted. I've never even been able to use tampons. When I finally got to see a gynecologist and she examined me, the pain was just indescribable. It was utter torture. I couldn't see what she was doing, but she told me after the exam that all she had done was gently touch the vagina entrance [vestibule] with a cotton Q-tip." Andrea, who suffered with the pain of PVD for ten years, said that the feel of a penis on her genitalia felt like "a bad blister being rubbed against the back of your heel." Another woman described the pain of penetration as feeling like the man had "spikes on his penis."

As with generalized vulvodynia (see Chapter 5), there are many different causes of PVD, all of which we discuss later in this chapter. The good news is that we have developed an algorithm to

YOUR BRAIN AND PVD

Can you "see" PVD in a woman's brain? That's just what I (Caroline) and my associates set out to discover in a series of studies looking at the brains of women with PVD and those without. In one study, we compared the total gray-matter volume and regional gray-matter densities in the brains of fourteen women with PVD and fourteen women without using a special type of MRI called brain voxel-based morphometry. We found that women with PVD had more gray matter in areas related to pain and stress. We also found that there was some relationship between certain areas of the brain and clinical symptoms, such as heightened pain sensitivity and increased pain catastrophizing.[2] In another study using functional MRI, which shows which parts of the brain are activated when you perform certain tasks or think about certain things, we found that the brains of women with PVD showed increased activation in regions associated with pain and sensation. The activation was similar to that seen in people with other chronic pain conditions, such as fibromyalgia and irritable bowel syndrome.[3]

From these studies, we learned that there appear to be changes in both the structure and function of the brains of women with PVD, particularly in the areas of pain processing. We're not sure yet how these processes change with treatment; those studies were still ongoing when we were writing this book. In the meantime, this is one of many reasons we recommend getting your pain identified and treated as quickly as possible. The longer the pain continues, the more likely such brain changes are to occur.

help you determine which of these likely plays a role in your pain (see Figure 6.1 on pages 82 and 83). It will also help you pick the appropriate treatment based on your specific profile.

Now, before we go on, we have a few things to say about our philosophy regarding PVD. For the last twenty-five years, very well-regarded experts in the field have treated PVD as if there were only two possible causes: inflammation or nerve damage. For years, some of the best vulvar specialists in the world treated women with steroids for inflammation or with antidepressants for damaged nerves. In fact, the world-renowned vulvar specialist Stanley Marinoff, MD, who was also my mentor, taught me (Andrew) this very approach.

Over the last ten years, however, well-done research on PVD has shattered such long-held beliefs about the origins of PVD. For instance, we found that women who took hormonal contraceptives were much more likely to have PVD. (This was probably the most important myth debunked since most of us were taught that oral contraceptives had nothing to do with the condition.) Other researchers showed that women with PVD had too many nerve endings in the vestibule and that relaxing the muscles of the pelvic floor improved pain in women with PVD. It soon became obvious that we weren't treating one disease but several underlying conditions that resulted in a similar set of symptoms.

At the same time that our understanding of the underlying pathology of the disease increased, so, too, did our treatment options. When I (Andrew) started treating PVD in the late 1990s, we had three treatments to offer women: interferon injections (to reduce inflammation), biofeedback to relax the muscles that surround the vestibule, and surgery to remove the overly sensitive tissue of the vestibule (vulvar vestibulectomy). Within the first five years of the new century, the treatment repertoire had expanded exponentially to include a variety of options.

However, we still didn't have a great strategy for choosing one treatment over another. The resulting hit-or-miss approach could take months, even years. Thus, we began looking at how we could use our patients' medical history and findings from their physical examinations and lab tests to distinguish among the different causes of PVD and target our treatment.

Vestibulodynia

The pain is confined to the vestibule: It (generally) stops outside of Hart's Line and there is (generally) no pain inside the vagina.

The pain is throughout the entire vestibule. (If the pain is significantly worse in the back part of the vestibule, consider a dual diagnosis and follow the next decision tree to the right as well.)

Hormonally Mediated Vestibulodynia

The pain began while:

- Taking hormonal contraceptive or other medications that affect hormones such as medications for endometriosis, breast cancer, acne, or infertility.
- After removal of ovaries.
- During breast feeding or menopause, or lack of a regular menstrual cycle.

There is a low calculated free testosterone.

May be associated with decreased libido, decreased arousal, decreased energy, or depression.

Congenital Neuroproliferative Vestibulodynia

There has always been pain (since first tampon insertion or first attempt at intercourse).

There has never been completely pain-free sex.

There may be sensitivity (or pain) when pushing in on the belly-button as compared to the rest of the abdomen (this pain may radiate towards the vagina).

Acquired Neuroproliferative Vestibulodynia

The pain began after:

- A severe allergic reaction to a topical medication.
- Severe yeast infection.

Women with a history of having very sensitive skin or many irritant or allergic reactions. May have abnormal genes including IL-1RA, MBL.

Desquamative Inflammation Vaginitis (DIV)

Thick, yellowish discharge that dries like glue, ruins underwear.

pH >5.0, many white blood cells and parabasal cells on wet mount.

FIGURE 6.1

The pain is much worse at 4, 6, and 8 o'clock position of the vestibule (and there is minimal or no pain on either side of the urethra).

There may be tenderness with deep pressure when applied to the perineum.

The pain is mainly in the vestibule but there is irritation, redness, and (possibly) fissures on the perineum or in the interlabial sulci.

Ulcers or erosions that may be confined to the vestibule but also may occur on the labia and perineum.

Hypertonic Pelvic Floor Dysfunction

The muscles of the pelvic floor are tight and tender (on exam by an experienced doctor or physical therapist).

There is an abnormal EMG of the pelvic floor muscles.

Vaginitis

Inflammation that includes the vestibule and vaginal mucosa. The vaginal mucosa typically looks inflamed and there is frequently yellowish discharge.

Bacterial vaginosis does not cause enough inflammation to cause vestibulodynia.

Lichen Planus

Ulceration in the vestibule that can have "fern-like" or violet borders. The erosions can extend into the vagina and can also affect the mouth. Very significant scarring of the vulva and vagina is possible.

Lichen Sclerosus

Ulcerations in the vestibule and on the labia but not in the vagina. Thick, white, itchy skin with very significant scarring.

Allergic Vaginitis

Semen allergy: swollen and inflamed vagina and vestibule. Does not happen if condom is used.

Latex or spermicide allergy: swollen and inflamed vagina and vestibule. Only occurs if condoms are used.

Candidiasis

Recurrent: Culture positive yeast infections that do not respond to three doses of fluconazole.

The chart we developed is the result (see Figure 6.1). As our explanations below show, we also developed our own terminology to better describe the various types of PVD. Your doctor probably won't recognize the terms we use—yet. We hope that they will eventually become the norm. In the meantime, we suggest that you bring this book to your visit to ensure that you and your doctor are on the same page.

UNDERLYING CAUSES AND TREATMENT OF PROVOKED VESTIBULODYNIA

Hormonally Mediated Vestibulodynia

This tongue-twisting condition has its roots in hormones. Recall that the opening of the vagina, the vulvar vestibule, requires adequate levels of both estrogen and testosterone to remain healthy. Yet, medications—particularly hormonal contraceptives, such as oral birth control pills, the contraceptive ring, the contraceptive patch, and contraceptive injections—often alter the levels of one or both. One study suggests that women who use hormonal contraception are more than six times as likely to develop PVD as those who have never used it.[4]

Obviously, only a small percentage of women (probably 1 to 3 percent) who take oral contraceptives develop PVD. Why this is, we don't know. It could have something to do with the type of contraception used. One study found that women who used low-dose birth control pills such as Lo-estrin were much more likely to develop PVD than women who used pills higher in estrogen, such as Ortho 1–35 or Ovcon-35.[5]

I (Irwin) have studied extensively the effects of estrogen and testosterone on the structure and function of genital tissues, so here's why. Oral contraceptive pills contain synthetic hormones similar to estrogen and progesterone. When you take the pill, your body assumes that it is getting enough of both hormones, so it signals your ovaries to suppress their own production of each. Since you are not producing your own natural hormones, hormone receptors in the vaginal and vulvar area also shut down. The end result is less estrogen available to cells than if you weren't taking the pills. If you take low-dose estrogen pills, that amount is even smaller.

In addition, hormonal contraceptives cause the liver to increase production of a protein called sex hormone binding globulin (SHBG). This protein attaches itself to testosterone in the blood, rendering the testosterone inactive. Therefore, the higher the SHBG, the lower the amount of active (or "free") testosterone. Since normal levels of free testosterone are required for a healthy vestibule, low levels of free testosterone can make the mucosa thin and painful.

In our experience, some of the newer birth control pills reduce free testosterone levels more than older brands, likely because of the type of synthetic progesterone they contain. Women on these pills seem to develop PVD at a higher rate than women on older pills. Plus, some women who use continuous contraception (so they can have fewer periods—once a year, in some cases) also seem to develop PVD at a higher rate. Other medications that can cause hormonally mediated vestibulodynia include those for infertility, endometriosis, and breast cancer. Removal of the ovaries, or oophorectomy, which puts a woman into sudden menopause, and menopause itself, when the ovaries shut down most of their production of estrogen, can also lead to hormonally mediated vestibulodynia.

The condition itself occurs gradually, with a sense of dryness, or inability to lubricate, often being the first sign. The hormonal changes might also lead to reduced desire (libido) and arousal even before any pain occurs. Clinically, hormonally mediated vestibulodynia results in tenderness of the entire vestibule. When your doctor conducts the cotton swab test we discussed in Chapter 3, the pain or burning occurs immediately inside Hart's Line. In addition, the tissue around the urethra, as well as in the back of the vestibule, is also tender. However, the tenderness stops immediately inside the vagina. Finally, the vestibular mucosa is usually dry and thin, appearing whitish with some overlying redness instead of its normal pink color.

If your doctor or you suspect hormonal causes behind your PVD, you should have your blood levels tested for estradiol, total testosterone, SHBG, and albumin. The last three levels are used to determine a "calculated free testosterone," that is, the amount of testosterone not bound to proteins in the blood and therefore active in the body. In a study I (Irwin) performed among nurses in our hospital with and without sexual dysfunction, we found that if you're between eighteen and thirty years old, your calculated free testosterone should be between 0.6 ng/dl and 1.0 ng/dl (where ng/dl stands for nanograms per deciliter). Women older than thirty should have levels between 0.4 ng/dl and 0.6 ng/dl. If either the estradiol or calculated free testosterone is low, your doctor should suspect hormonally mediated vestibulodynia. (We don't give a number for estrogen levels because they vary greatly throughout the menstrual cycle and even throughout the day. As women get older, their average estrogen levels drop, but they have higher peaks and deeper troughs, which probably account for the fibroids and hot flashes women experience during these years.)

Treating Hormonally Mediated Vestibulodynia
If medications that affect hormones are behind your problem, you need to stop taking or using them. Doctors sometimes think that applying hormonal creams to the vulvar area will solve the problem, but they won't if you're still taking the medications. Remember: Your body has shut down estrogen and testosterone receptors in those areas. The hormones from the cream simply can't get into cells to do their work.

Typically, your estradiol level should return to normal within a month of stopping hormonal contraceptives. However, the calculated free testosterone often remains persistently low. Some research suggests levels may remain low for months or even years.[6] That's where hormonal creams or gels come into play. I (Andrew) recommend a combination gel containing estradiol and testosterone, which you can have made at a compounding pharmacy (see "What Is a Compounding Pharmacy?"). I (Irwin) recommend local estradiol and systemic testosterone.

Be patient. It may take at least six weeks before you see any improvement. Even after three months, your pain may only improve by one-third to one-half. It typically takes four to six months to recover completely. We recommend that every woman whose PVD developed while she was using hormonal contraceptives or any medication that affects hormone levels be treated for hormonally mediated vestibulodynia for at least three months before considering other treatments.

WHAT IS A COMPOUNDING PHARMACY?

Some treatments your doctor prescribes, such as topical gabapentin cream or the estradiol-testosterone gel we recommend for women who have been taking birth control pills, you may need to order from a compounding pharmacy. These pharmacies can custom-mix medications based on nonstandard dosages or with different nonactive ingredients (such as the gel) than the standard prescription. Your doctor should be able to recommend a reputable compounding pharmacy in your area.

Hypertonic Pelvic Floor Muscle Dysfunction

This condition, also called levator ani syndrome or vaginismus, is another common cause of PVD. In this condition, the muscles that compose the floor of the pelvis and come together in the back part of the vestibule—the pubococcygeus, puborectalis, and transverse perineal muscles—become tight and tender (see Figure 6.2). When these muscles are tight, less blood flows through them, providing less oxygen to cells and resulting in a build up of lactic acid. The lactic acid causes the sensations of burning, rawness, throbbing, stabbing, and aching so many women experience. In addition, it causes severe tenderness and redness of the vestibule near the perineum.

Any doctor or physical therapist who knows how to examine these muscles should be able to diagnose this condition. During the exam, the doctor or therapist should gently push on these muscles to see if they are tight, tender, weak, or inflexible. There might also be trigger points, that is, very tender knots of muscle.

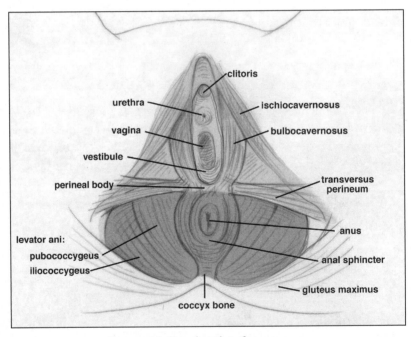

FIGURE 6.2 Female pelvic floor anatomy

Two other tests, electromyography and perineometry, both described in more detail in Chapter 13, can confirm the diagnosis and measure the muscle tightness. Women with pelvic floor dysfunction (PFD) often also have urinary symptoms such as frequency, urgency, and incomplete emptying of the bladder. In addition, constipation, hemorrhoids, and rectal fissures (tears in the anal area) are common. Finally, women may also have low back, hip pain, or both.

Treating Pelvic Floor Muscle Dysfunction

The most important treatment for PFD is pelvic floor physical therapy performed by a qualified women's health physical therapist. You can find one in your area through the American Physical Therapists Association website (www.womenshealthapta.org). In a study that I (Caroline) and my associates conducted, we found that eight sessions of this therapy reduced pain sensitivity and intensity, increased sexual function, and decreased pain anxiety and catastrophizing thoughts.[7] Even more importantly, when examining the specific effects of this therapy on the pelvic floor, we found normal measures of pelvic floor function. We discuss physical therapy in more detail in Chapter 13.

Other treatments include biofeedback, heat therapy, muscle relaxants such as compounded diazepam (Valium) vaginal suppositories, and Botox injections into the muscles itself. All of these, however, are in addition to, not instead of, the physical therapy.

Neuroproliferative Vestibulodynia

In this condition, women have an increased number of nerve endings called c-afferent nociceptors in their vestibular mucosa, sometimes up to ten times as many as women without PVD. When these c-afferent nociceptors fire, the brain translates these signals into the sensations of burning, rawness, and cutting. That's why women

MEDICAL HYPNOTHERAPY FOR PROVOKED VESTIBULODYNIA

Although we'd certainly not recommend it on its own, medical hypnosis can be a valuable adjunct to the treatments described here for PVD. When I (Caroline) and my team tested hypnosis on eight women with PVD, their pain and sex lives significantly improved after just six sessions.[8] Hypnosis is a trancelike state in which you're more open to suggestions (to experience more control over your pain, for example). Because of this openness, you're better able to change your perceptions and understanding related to the pain. We think this change in thinking helps dampen the level of the pain signals coming from the brain.

with this form of PVD feel as if they are being "cut with a hot knife" during sexual penetration. In fact, women with this condition may be so hypersensitive in the vestibule that they feel intense pain with only the slightest pressure (e.g., that of a cotton swab).

So, how do women develop increased nerve endings in the vestibule? Research suggests two ways: They are either born with the condition, or it develops as a result of chronic yeast infections or a severe allergic reaction (often to an antifungal cream or even a partner's semen).[9]

As you learned in Chapter 1, the tissue of the vulvar vestibule is embryologically derived from tissue called the urogenital ridge, also called the primitive urogenital sinus. Only two other places in the body also have tissue derived from the primitive urogenital sinus: the urethra and, in some women, the inside of the umbilicus, or belly button. We and our colleagues conducted a research study that showed that some women with primary neuroproliferative vestibulodynia were almost as sensitive in their belly buttons as at their vestibules.[10] They hated being touched there. In addition, in some women the discomfort they felt when we touched in the um-

IMPROVING THE COTTON SWAB TEST

While the cotton swab test seems relatively simple, the results depend on where the doctor touches and how the doctor touches (rolling, stroking, or palpating, using soft or strong force). Some clinicians use a wet swab (as we recommend), others a dry swab. These variations can confound diagnosis in both community and research settings.[11]

That's why I (Caroline) invented a new instrument called a vulvalgesiometer. I know, the name of the device is very long and hard to say, but I was not sure what to call it when I first made it. An algesiometer is something that measures pain, and I added the "vulv" to indicate that it was for use in the vulva (although it can be used anywhere on the body). It is a simple device consisting of a set of handheld pen-like devices with springs calibrated at various compression rates. A cotton swab extends from the end of the device. The vulvalgesiometer provides prespecified levels of force and thus a standard way to evaluate a woman's pain threshold.[12] Currently used mainly in research settings, it may eventually find its way into gynecology and urology offices. I am also working on a fancier version of this device that will cut down on time!

bilicus radiated toward the vagina.[13] So, if you have pain in your vestibule *and* in your belly button, we think that's proof that you were born with congenital neuroproliferative vestibulodynia.

Now, onto women who develop it later in life. Researchers at Cornell University have showed that some women with PVD have genetic changes that limit their body's ability to turn down inflammation or overcome yeast infections. This explains why so many women with PVD report that their symptoms began after a yeast infection.[14] The infection triggers the release of immune cells called mast cells; these in turn release a chemical called nerve growth factor, which can trigger the growth of new nerve endings.[15] Normally, once the infection clears, the inflammatory reaction turns off. In some women, however, it keeps going, leading to the nerve over-growth that is the hallmark of this form of the disease.

Treating Neuroproliferative Vestibulodynia

If we catch the condition early enough, we inject a medication into the vestibule called interferon-alpha, which inhibits mast cell activity.[16] However, the injections only work if used within the first few months of the onset of symptoms, before the growth of new nerve endings. Other options include the following:

- Topical anesthetics. The goal here is to numb the nociceptors. To that end, we often recommend that women apply topical anesthetics such as lidocaine before sex. There's also some evidence that applying lidocaine frequently throughout the day and at night (by putting a cotton ball soaked with 5 percent lidocaine in the vaginal opening and leaving it there overnight) can reduce the pain.[17]

- Antidepressants and antiseizure drugs. Another approach is to reduce the signals traveling through the nerves of the central nervous system (the spinal cord and brain), thus reducing the pain. Tricyclic antidepressants (amitriptyline, nortriptyline, desipramine), the selective norepinephrine reuptake inhibitor antidepressants (SNRIs) venlafaxine (Effexor) and duloxetine (Cymbalta), and antiepileptic drugs such as gabapentin (Neurontin), pregabalin (Lyrica), and topiramate (Topamax) can help. Another option that's been showing success is compounding the antiepileptic medications into a cream. This lets you apply the medication directly to the vestibule to limit side effects.[18]

The medications should be started at a low dose and increased weekly until the PVD is at least 75 percent better (or the side effects are too great). Side effects include sleepiness, dry mouth, constipation, palpitations, and weight gain with the tricyclic anti-depressants; insomnia, nausea, decreased libido, and difficulty achieving orgasm with the SNRIs, as well as withdrawal reactions if you try to stop taking them on your own; and headache, lethargy, and difficulty thinking clearly with the antiseizure medications.

One problem we frequently see with new patients is that they were started on one of these medications, but their dosage was never increased. Or they were given the wrong type of antidepressant, such as a selective serotonin reuptake inhibitor (e.g., Prozac or Paxil), which doesn't seem to help with PVD.

- Capsaicin cream. Capsaicin is the substance that gives chili peppers their heat. When applied to the vestibule, the cream causes severe burning because it stimulates the release of substance P, one of the body's neurotransmitters for pain and heat. However, with chronic exposure (we have our patients apply the cream for twenty minutes nightly for six to twelve weeks), the nerve endings become depleted of substance P, resulting in far less vestibular pain. If you stop applying the cream, however, the nerve endings will "recharge" and again be capable of feeling pain. So you may need to use the cream indefinitely.

Surgery: A Very Successful Option

The final treatment is surgery, called vulvar vestibulectomy with vaginal advancement. It involves removing about a postage-stamp-sized piece of tissue from vestibule, thereby reducing the number of nerve endings. A four-page illustration of this surgery can be found on our website (www.cvvd.org/publications), and photographs of the surgery may be found on the website of the Institute for Sexual Medicine (http://sexualmed.org).

We recommend surgery as a first option, however, only for women with primary neuroproliferative vestibulodynia, the belly

button type. That's because we have found over the years that
medical approaches like those described above simply don't work
very well in these women. Women with secondary neuroproliferative vestibulodynia, the type that occurs after a period of pain-free
sex, should, however, try several of the medical approaches described above before considering surgery.

Kathy, a patient of ours who had primary neuroproliferative
vestibulodynia, spent eight years with vulvar pain, saw at least fifteen different doctors, and tried dozens of treatments. Nothing
worked, and none of the doctors suggested surgery until she found
me. I immediately recommended the vestibulectomy. "Up until
recently, my partner and I had intercourse only very, very rarely,"
Kathy said. "I always had pain: sometimes horrible, unbearable
pain. Since the surgery and recovery, we are now having intercourse regularly, and it doesn't hurt."

The procedure itself is typically performed on an outpatient basis under spinal or conscious sedation. The main complication is
decreased lubrication, which occurs in about a quarter of women
undergoing the procedure. Overall, however, the success rate is
excellent. In one study of 104 women that I (Andrew) published
in *The Journal of Sexual Medicine*, 93 percent said they were satisfied or very satisfied with the surgical outcome, and 87 percent
said their sex lives improved after surgery. That's pretty dramatic,
given that 74 percent of the women were completely unable to
have intercourse prior to surgery, and only 7 percent had had intercourse two or more times a month. After surgery, 89 percent of
the women said they were having sex, 56 percent of them three or
more times a month! When we asked the women, "In retrospect,
knowing what you know now about the surgery, would you have it
again?" 93 percent said yes. The same number also said that they
would recommend the vestibulectomy to another woman with
similar symptoms.

We also saw very low rates of complication with these women. One woman developed a blood clot that had to be drained immediately after surgery, and two had Bartholin's gland cysts from the surgery that had to be treated.[19] Recently, I (Andrew) completed a similar study on an additional 110 women. Nearly all (99 percent) said they would have the surgery again.

If you do decide to undergo surgery, please keep several things in mind. First, choose your surgeon very carefully. You should look for one who has performed this procedure many times. As it is not a very common one, you may need to travel to find an experienced surgeon. You can contact an academic medical center or the National Vulvodynia Association to try to locate an experienced surgeon. Once you have found one, it is important to have a consultation to see if you feel comfortable with him or her. Remember, it is not rude to ask a potential surgeon how many of these surgeries he or she has performed. Ask about the surgeon's success rate, how he or she defines success, and whether he or she has published this success rate in a peer-reviewed medical journal. In addition, you should ask the surgeon how he or she determines what tissue and how much to remove. We (Andrew and Irwin) strongly believe that the mucosa of the entire vestibule should be removed, not just the tissue in the back part. Some surgeons do "pain mapping" and remove only the most painful areas, which tend to be located in the back. However, this means that the less painful areas then become the most painful.

Finally, keep in mind that complete recovery typically takes at least six weeks, and it will be several months before you can begin having sex.

Vaginitis

Vaginitis is inflammation of the vagina. There are two categories: infectious and sterile (noninfectious). Sometimes, although fairly rarely, the inflammation may be so severe that inflammatory white blood cells pour out of the vagina and coat the vestibule, leading to inflammation of the vestibule (i.e., vestibulitis) and PVD.

The two types of infectious vaginitis that are inflammatory enough to cause PVD are yeast (candidiasis) and trichomoniasis (see Chapter 7). Other bacterial infections of the vagina, such as bacterial vaginosis and Gardnerella, do not cause enough inflammation to lead to PVD. And even yeast infections rarely lead to PVD.

Sterile vaginitis can be caused by an irritant or allergic reaction to chemicals such as vaginal antifungal creams, spermicides, lubricants, and latex in condoms or sex toys. In addition, sterile vaginitis can be caused by a lack of estrogen like that described in the section on hormonally mediated vestibulodynia or by a condition called desquamative inflammatory vaginitis (DIV).

The characteristic sign of DIV is a copious yellowish discharge that dries like glue on the vulva or underwear. If you looked at this discharge under a microscope, you'd see sheets of white blood cells and many immature cells of the vagina called parabasal cells. Unfortunately, we don't know what causes DIV. One theory holds that a lack of estrogen is behind the condition—that the tremendous inflammation destroys normal cells, leaving only immature cells.

Finally, an allergic reaction to your partner's semen can lead to vaginitis. A clue that this is behind your pain is if you have no problems when your partner uses a condom but experience severe swelling and irritation if he doesn't.

Clinically, when PVD is caused by vaginitis, there is redness and tenderness in both the vagina and vestibule (whereas in other types of PVD, the vagina is spared), heavy yellowish discharge that causes inflammation at the vestibule, and a large increase in the number of white blood cells when the discharge is examined under the microscope. So, even if yeast is present under the microscope, without the concurrent white blood cells, the yeast infection is probably not the cause of your PVD pain. Unfortunately, most women with PVD have been unnecessarily subjected to numerous courses of antibiotics and antifungals that do nothing to resolve the pain. (For more on the different types of vaginitis and their treatments, see Chapter 7.)

WHAT ABOUT A LOW OXALATE DIET?

We hear from many women who believe that a diet low in oxalate-containing foods will improve their PVD. Oxalates are naturally occurring molecules found in most plant-based foods such as soy, fruit, and chocolate. They can bind with calcium to form calcium oxalate, the primary cause of kidney stones. But there is no evidence to implicate them in vulvodynia. A 1997 study evaluating women with PVD who followed a low-oxalate diet found just 10 percent were able to resume pain-free sex,[20] while a later study found no difference in terms of painful sex between women with PVD who followed such a diet and those who didn't.[21]

The largest study on the topic was published in 2008. The authors evaluated the diets of 242 women with PVD and 242 without from nine communities around Boston. They found no difference in terms of the amount of high-oxalate foods either group ate and no increased risk of developing vulvodynia in the women who ate a high-oxalate diet.[22] Bottom line: Worry about the amount of fat, calories, and sodium in your diet, not oxalates.

THREE SIMPLE CONVERSATIONS: DR. ANDREW GOLDSTEIN GIVES CREDIT WHERE CREDIT IS DUE

Sometimes a brief conversation can have the greatest impact on your life. I learned this one sunny spring day seven years ago, when I was attending the second National Institutes of Health conference on vulvodynia. While I certainly found many of the lectures given that day informative, none offered information that would significantly change how I was treating my patients with vulvodynia.

(continues)

THREE SIMPLE CONVERSATIONS: DR. ANDREW GOLDSTEIN GIVES CREDIT WHERE CREDIT IS DUE

(continued)

However, when walking to lunch, I saw Gordon Davis, MD, one of the world's leading vulvar specialists. Dr. Davis, who lives in Phoenix, had had quite an eventful trip to Maryland. When he arrived, he developed severe abdominal pain, went straight to the hospital, and underwent an emergency procedure. After he assured me that he was fine, we started discussing the conference, and he asked what he'd missed.

"Gordon, I am both confused and excited about the conference," I told him. "We've heard lectures that certain genetic defects allow increased inflammation, which may cause vestibulodynia. Another lecture discussed an increased density of nerve endings in women with vestibulodynia. Another lecture discussed the risk of infection and vestibulodynia. I am just not sure how I can put it all together."

Dr. Davis looked up, smiled, and said, "Andrew, just get them off the [birth control] pill and give them estrogen cream." Now, I have to admit that I was younger then, and with this youth came a bit of arrogance. I rolled my eyes and replied, "Sure, Gordon."

"Just try it on ten women and see," he said.

Since I had great respect for Dr. Davis, I gave it a try. Amazingly, over the next few months, I tried this relatively easy intervention on my patients with vestibulodynia, and the pain improved dramatically in about half.

About six months later I was at another conference. This time I was talking to Irwin, and I mentioned the connection between oral contraceptives and vestibulodynia, and he mentioned that his lab had recently shown that the vestibule has a very high density of testosterone receptors. Since oral contraceptives reduce testosterone, it made sense that oral contraceptives could cause vestibulodynia by lowering testosterone receptors.

He suggested that I use testosterone on my patients with vestibulodynia. So over the next few months, I tried the combination

(continues)

(*continued*)

of estrogen and testosterone on my patients, and I was amazed with the results: About two-thirds got completely better!

I would be remiss were I to leave out a third conversation. The following year I was introduced to Susan Kellogg, PhD, a gynecologic nurse practitioner and sexologist. We sat at large table during the lunch break of the annual meeting of the International Society for the Study of Women's Sexual Health. I am bit foggy on the exact specifics of the conversation but the take-home message was that if I wasn't using pelvic floor physical therapy as part of the treatment for vestibulodynia, I was missing the boat. And you know what? She was absolutely right!

BOTTOM LINE

We believe that it is imperative for any woman who thinks she has PVD to undergo a thorough evaluation by a physician or a nurse practitioner. Even if your health-care professional is not familiar with all the causes of vestibular pain, together you can use the diagnostic algorithm provided in this chapter to determine the cause(s) of your pain. Then you can use a targeted treatment approach for your type of PVD. In this way you can avoid unnecessary treatments and more quickly find the correct solution for your pain.

The two chapters you've just read address the two most common causes of painful sex. However, they are far from the only causes, as you'll see in the rest of Part II. It's also important to keep in mind that you may have more than one underlying cause of your dyspareunia. Remember my (Andrew's) patient Kathy who had the surgery? While the pain in her vulvar area stopped after the surgery, she still had pain near her urethra. It turns out she had interstitial cystitis, a condition you'll learn about in Chapter 9. After treatment for the interstitial cystitis, she is now pain-free in all areas. So, don't skip the next chapters just because you think you've figured out your problem!

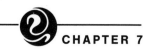
Could It Be an Infection?

As we began writing this chapter, the Centers for Disease Control and Prevention (CDC) had just released a report noting that one in six Americans is infected with herpes simplex virus type 2 (HSV-2), or herpes. Herpes is an incurable sexually transmitted infection that can cause recurrent and painful genital sores. Women are particularly at risk, with one in five women affected, and nearly half of all African American women.[1] One of the main worries about herpes infection is that it nearly triples the risk of HIV infection. For the purposes of this book, however, we want to focus on another implication: its contribution to painful sex.

Herpes is just one of numerous infections, sexually transmitted or otherwise, that may be causing your sexual pain. Even if they don't cause the pain directly, some infections, such as yeast (candidiasis) and bacterial vaginosis (BV), increase your risk of provoked vestibulodynia (PVD). The good news is that, unlike with PVD and other underlying causes of dyspareunia, relief may be only a pill or tube of cream away.

SEXUALLY TRANSMITTED INFECTIONS

Herpes

There are actually two types of herpes: herpes simplex virus type 1 (HSV-1) and HSV-2. While people typically think that HSV-1 causes cold sores on the mouth and HSV-2 causes genital lesions, that's not always the case. As oral sex has become more prevalent, the rates of HSV-1 infections on the vulva and HSV-2 infections on the mouth have increased.

Once you're infected with the herpes virus, you're infected for life. The virus lives in your nerves. It is usually dormant, but when your immune system is suppressed—due to stress, hormonal changes, or other infections—the virus is reactivated, resulting in an outbreak.

The classic herpes lesion is a grapelike cluster of small pimples that pop, causing open sores. Herpes typically only causes pain in one area and almost never on both sides of the vulva at the same time. However, the lesions can appear anywhere on your genitals, from the inner folds of your labia and clitoral area to your outer thighs and anal area—even on your butt! The pain can be severe and constant, particularly when you urinate or have a bowel movement, or it may occur only during sex. Keep in mind that even if you don't have any visible vulvar lesions, you might still have an active infection that you can pass on to your partner because you may have lesions in your vagina.

Many women get what we call a "prodrome" before an outbreak. You may feel some itching, tingling, or even pain in the area in which lesions are about to erupt. Some women even report that their mood plummets, which could relate to the release of inflammatory chemicals as your immune system gears up to fight the virus.

Some women have pain even after the outbreak is over; this is called postherpetic neuralgia. Sometimes postherpetic neuralgia can cause pain in the clitoris; this is called clitorodynia. The typical symptoms of clitorodynia include a burning, gnawing pain confined to the clitoris.

Diagnosis. If you suspect you might have herpes but have never been formally diagnosed, see your doctor immediately. Taking a culture of the sore during an active outbreak is the best way to confirm the diagnosis. A diagnosis is important because today there are several medications you can take both to prevent outbreaks and, if they threaten, to stop them in their tracks. This can also prevent transmission to your partner.

Treatment. Treatment includes the antivirals acyclovir (Zovirax), valacyclovir (Valtrex), and famciclovir (Famvir). Sometimes, if you have frequent outbreaks, you can take these medications prophylactically (i.e., before an outbreak) on a daily basis to prevent an outbreak and to decrease the risk of transmission to a partner. Side effects are typically very mild but include headache, flu-like symptoms, nausea, vomiting, reduced appetite, and joint pain. It is most important to start treatment within the first thirty-six hours of an outbreak.

Some studies suggest that the supplements L-lysine and zinc, both available in health food stores and many drugstores, may also reduce herpes outbreaks. Nonprescription drug treatments that can help include sitz baths and over-the-counter pain medications. Just make sure always to follow label directions when taking such products; acetaminophen (Tylenol) and ibuprofen (Motrin) might seem benign, but too much can fry your liver or have other dangerous effects.

Pelvic Inflammatory Disease

Untreated gonorrhea or chlamydia, two other common sexually transmitted diseases, can lead to pelvic inflammatory disease (PID), a common cause of pelvic pain and deep dyspareunia (for more on deep dyspareunia, see Chapter 9). The condition, which affects about 1 million women per year, occurs as the bacteria that cause these diseases make their way from the vagina and cervix to the upper reproductive tract, affecting the fallopian tubes, uterus, and pelvic cavity. PID can cause adhesions (scarring), an ectopic (tubal) pregnancy, bowel obstructions, pelvic pain, fallopian tube abscesses, and even infection of the abdominal/pelvic cavity itself (peritonitis).

About one woman in three with PID develops chronic pelvic pain, pain during intercourse with deep thrusting, or both. Unfortunately, rates of both chlamydia and gonorrhea are on the rise in the United States, with chlamydia responsible for about 40 percent of all cases of PID. Approximately 10 percent of college-age women have chlamydia at any given time.

Symptoms of PID include pain in your lower abdomen that gets worse during sex; abnormal vaginal bleeding, such as after sex and between your periods; pain during or after sex that occurs deep within your pelvic region; yellowish vaginal or cervical discharge; and, in some women, fever and/or painful urination. Severe cases may lead to the development of adhesions (scar tissue) between organs in the abdominal/pelvic cavity. Adhesions are a primary reason for the deep dyspareunia many women experience with PID. In addition, adhesions are also common after surgery. They are your body's way of reacting to trauma of any kind to the peritoneum (the tissue that lines the abdominal cavity). Adhesions are a common cause of pelvic pain because the peritoneum is rich in nerve fibers, and nerves, you recall, transmit pain signals.

In addition, adhesions caused by PID can cause scarring of your fallopian tubes, leading to infertility or ectopic (tubal) pregnancy.

Diagnosis. Diagnosing PID is challenging, given that no single test is available. Instead, your doctor arrives at the diagnosis based on your symptoms, the appearance of your reproductive tract, and tests for gonorrhea and chlamydia. The gold standard for diagnosis is a surgical procedure called laparoscopy, in which a camera is inserted through an incision in the belly button into the pelvic cavity to look for signs of infection.

Treatment. The primary treatment for PID is antibiotics to wipe out the infectious agents. Unfortunately, the primary antibiotics used to treat gonorrhea, called fluoroquinolones, are now often useless given the rise of resistant bacteria. Luckily, a variety of other antibiotics are still available, including doxycycline, ceftriaxone (Rocephin), cefoxitin (Mefoxin), and metronidazole (Flagyl), often in combination. Side effects vary based on the drug but include diarrhea, headache, loss of appetite, nausea, vaginal itching or discharge, swollen tongue or trouble swallowing (doxycycline), and sores or swelling in the genital or rectal area (doxycycline).

In cases of severe PID infection, you may need intravenous antibiotics before switching over to oral versions. You should also let your partner(s) know that you have PID. They should be tested for gonorrheal or chlamydial infection, even if they have no symptoms. If you have adhesions, your doctor may try to remove them surgically to relieve your pain and dyspareunia.[2]

Trichomoniasis

Trichomoniasis (frequently shortened to "trich") is one the most common sexually transmitted infections in the world, affecting up to 180 million people annually. In the United States, it affects about 3 percent of women, up to 13 percent of African American women, and a total of 3 to 5 million women per year.[3] Unlike herpes, which is caused by a virus, or gonorrhea, which is caused by bacteria, the trich culprit is a tiny protozoan called *Trichomonas vaginalis*. This little bugger can infect your vagina and urethra, as well as glands near the urethra and vaginal openings.

Common symptoms include itching, foul-smelling vaginal discharge (typically frothy yellowish green), and painful urination, as well as dyspareunia. Sound familiar? Most are also the symptoms of your plain vanilla yeast infection. Unfortunately, many women try to self-treat such symptoms with over-the-counter products, never realizing that not only will those attempts not help, but they may make the sexual pain worse.

Diagnosis. Your health-care professional should diagnose trich by examining your vaginal discharge under a microscope or performing a DNA probe of your vaginal discharge. Correct diagnosis is important since trich not only causes sexual pain but can damage your fallopian tubes (causing infertility), lead to preterm labor, and induce changes in cervical cells that can increase your risk of cancer.[4] The infection also increases your risk of contracting HIV.[5]

Treatment. First, stop having sex. There's no point in passing the infection back and forth between you and your partner. As with most sexually transmitted infections, both of you will need treatment. The infection is treated with the oral antibiotics tinidazole (Tindamax) or metronidazole (Flagyl). Side effects include nausea, loss of appetite, diarrhea, and headache. It is important that you not drink any alcohol within forty-eight hours of taking either of these antibiotics because it may cause severe nausea.

Continue abstaining from sex until at least one week after your final dose. Then get rechecked after your finish your course of drugs; if the infection hasn't cleared, you'll need more antibiotics, possibly at higher doses. The risk here is that continued courses of antibiotics could trigger a yeast infection (see "The Downside of Antibiotics").

Syphilis

We tend to think of syphilis as a disease from the days of yore when sailors pulled into port and consorted with prostitutes. And, indeed, the rate of syphilis in the United States reached an all-time low in 2000, low enough that the CDC actually put a plan in play to eliminate it entirely. Then the numbers began creeping up, with the rate of syphilis in women more than tripling just between 2007 and 2008.[6]

Syphilis is a bacterial infection. Like herpes, however, it also can cause genital ulcers. In fact, that's often the first clue that something's wrong. The ulcers generally appear about three weeks after infection. Another sign of infection, particularly of one that's been around a while, is enlarged and tender lymph nodes. If the infection continues, you may notice a rash on the palms of your hands and soles of your feet, as well as in your vaginal area. While not a common cause of sexual pain, the early-stage lesions of syphilis can hurt during intercourse. Plus, like most sexually transmitted infections, active infection with syphilis can be particularly dangerous to a fetus during pregnancy.

Diagnosis. In the past, the diagnosis of syphilis was made when a physician examined the discharge from the sores using a special "dark-field" microscope. However, a very inexpensive blood test

called a rapid plasma regain, or RPR, is now the easiest way to diagnosis syphilis.

Treatment. Syphilis is treated with antibiotics. It is important
that you (and your partner) get treatment since untreated syphilis
can affect your brain and central nervous system, as well as your
heart.

Candidiasis

> I got a bad sinus infection, and my doctor prescribed a powerful
> antibiotic. It ended up giving me a severe yeast infection, so she
> prescribed Monistat. After using it, I started having severe burn-
> ing in my vulvar area. I went back to her numerous times and
> each time was given different medications to take, either orally
> or vaginally. The burning increased to the point that I would work
> all day, and as soon as I got home, I would collapse on the living
> room floor screaming and crying because of the burning. I even
> tried putting plain yogurt on a pad and wearing that to bed. . . .
> The coolness felt good for at least a few minutes.
>
> After being in agonizing pain for over a year and visiting nu-
> merous gynecologists, I finally found Dr. Andrew Goldstein who,
> when I told him about the history of medications, told me that by
> "bombarding" me with so much medication in the vaginal area, I
> had caused an overgrowth of nerve endings in my vulva.
> —ROBIN, THIRTY-TWO

We can't tell you how many women tell us that their vulvar pain
began after a yeast infection or a series of them. Breanne told us
the story of what happened when she was twenty-three: "I had
been recovering from a yeast infection and had sex with my fi-

ancée, who was in town visiting me. My genital area started to burn soon after we started having sex." Since then, Breanne has been diagnosed with vestibulodynia and, after other treatments failed, is planning on surgery. Karla told us that her symptoms began with constant yeast infections, then "terrible daily irritation and painful sex." Marcy recalls visiting numerous doctors over the years, "all of whom looked for yeast infections or urinary tract infections to no avail."

THE DOWNSIDE OF ANTIBIOTICS

One reason life expectancy in this country has increased so significantly over the last fifty years is antibiotics. These seemingly magical drugs can wipe out bacteria like a sponge cleaning a dirty counter. Unfortunately, they take more of a "weapons of mass destruction" approach than a smart bomb approach, wiping out all bacteria, the good as well as the bad.

The thing is, your vaginal relies on good bacteria called lactobacilli to maintain normal pH. If the lactobacilli are killed by antibiotics, other organisms can take hold. Next thing you know, you have the familiar itchiness and discharge of a yeast infection.

Many women with dyspareunia report that their pain began just after a yeast infection and gets worse during yeast infections. In one study of 1,000 women, about 10 percent had symptoms of vulvodynia, and 35 percent of those women said they thought a yeast infection had caused their symptoms.[7] If you tend to get such infections while taking antibiotics, ask your doctor about a prescription for fluconazole (Diflucan), an antifungal that can reduce the risk of yeast infections.[8] Common side effects include nausea, vomiting, diarrhea or upset stomach, headache, dizziness, unusual or unpleasant taste in your mouth, and skin rash or itching. And skip the probiotics; unfortunately, there's no good evidence that these "good" bacteria work to prevent antibiotic-related yeast infections.[9]

We know that there is a strong link between a history of yeast infections and dyspareunia, not only from our own experience but from several published studies. In one such study of 301 women with vulvodynia, 64 percent reported a history of yeast infections.[10] Another found that women with vulvodynia were three times more likely to report a history of yeast infections than women without. A third study of women found that those with an active candida infection were nearly 1.5 times more likely to report painful sex than those without.[11]

Most yeast infections are caused by the *Candida albicans* fungus, although infection with other types of candida, particularly *Candida glabrata*, is increasing. Two other infections, trichomoniasis, covered earlier in the chapter, and bacterial vaginosis (discussed below) are often confused with one another, leading to high rates of misdiagnosis and incorrect or delayed treatments. Unlike trich, candida vaginitis is not usually transmitted sexually.

Experts estimate that about three out of every four women will have at least one bout of candida vaginitis before menopause; half of those women will have at least one more. Between 5 and 8 percent of women overall suffer from recurrent candida infections that often don't respond to single-dose treatments.[12]

Typical symptoms include a thick, cottage-cheesy discharge along with vaginal soreness, irritation, vulvar burning, dyspareunia, and painful urination. If you could look at your own labia and vulva, you'd see some swelling and redness, sometimes with some small lesions. Symptoms tend to get worse just before your period and improve during menstruation.

Even without any symptoms, your vagina may still have candida. One study found that between 15 and 20 percent of women had yeast in their vagina, even though they had no signs of infection.[13] Women who are pregnant, use birth control pills, or have uncontrolled diabetes are more likely to show signs of candida, as are postmenopausal women who use estrogen-replacement therapy. Experts suspect some type of hormonal link to the infection since high levels of estrogen create the kind of high-glucose environment in which sugar-loving candida thrive. About one in five cases result from the antibiotic use we discussed earlier, which wipes out "good" bacteria that help keep the vagina at a candida-repelling pH level.

The pain of candida comes as the fungi damage cells in the vaginal area, triggering inflammation, swelling, and redness as your vagina sheds cells from its lining. While the infection itself is painful, contributing to pain during intercourse (and at all other times), recurrent infections may trigger the type of nerve overgrowth that leads to PVD. Not only that, but each recurrent infection seems to hurt worse, regardless of its severity.

Diagnosis. Doctors should diagnose candida infections by examining vaginal secretions under a microscope (a wet mount) and measuring vaginal pH. However, these simple tests can lead to false negatives, delaying treatment. So, if your symptoms suggest candidiasis but the tests are negative, ask for a fungal culture to confirm. And make sure you get some type of test; too many women (and their doctors) try to diagnose yeast-based on symptoms and clinical appearance alone, which leads to high rates of misdiagnosis. One study found that women who thought they had a yeast infection were correct only 51 percent of the time. Another showed that doctors who relied only on an exam, without a wet mount or culture, were also wrong more than 20 percent of the time.[14]

Treatment. Don't try to treat your yeast infection on your own. Up to half of women who do this misdiagnose their infections and wind up treating the wrong thing. Numerous treatments are available for candida vaginitis, including antifungal creams, vaginal

tablets, suppositories, and even coated tampons. Most yeast infections are easy to treat, with "cure" rates ranging between 80 and
90 percent, depending on the severity.

More doctors these days are trying to cure yeast infections with
high doses of topical antifungal creams used for a very short period.
However, this doesn't seem to work as well for women with severe,
complicated vaginitis, which may require treatment for up to two
weeks or even several months. In addition, these high-dose creams
can be very irritating, especially in women susceptible to allergic
reactions or increased inflammation.

Thus, we generally prefer to use oral antifungals such as itra-
conazole (Sporanox) or fluconazole (Diflucan) instead of the topical antifungals. If your infection doesn't seem to respond to typical
treatments, ask your doctor to identify the type of yeast infection.
Candida glabrata vaginitis often doesn't improve with typical antifungals and may require vaginal capsules of boric acid or flucyto-
sine cream. In some instances, you may need a steroidal cream as
well as an antifungal cream to cool the inflammation.

Women with recurrent yeast infections might want to get
checked for diabetes, since uncontrolled diabetes—with its high

BLAME IT ON YOUR GENES

Scientists at Cornell University have found that women with
PVD are more likely to have an abnormal form of one of several
different genes. One is for a protein called mannose-binding
lectin, which is part of the body's immune system. If you have a
broken form of this gene, you are more likely to get yeast infections. In addition, they have found that defects in other genes that
are supposed to limit inflammation in the body increase the risk
of PVD. So, if you are susceptible to recurrent yeast infections
or prone to increased inflammations, you are at greater risk for
dyspareunia.

blood-glucose levels—is a known contributor. Corticosteroids and other immune suppressants are also risk factors for recurrent yeast infections. To prevent recurrences, talk to your doctor about prophylactic therapy with weekly doses of oral antifungals or weekly use of an oral antifungal suppository to suppress fungal levels.

Bacterial Vaginosis

We want to discuss bacterial vaginosis (BV) briefly because many of the patients who come to our office have been told that their sexual pain is caused by BV. However, in our experience, BV is not a cause of long-term dyspareunia.

BV occurs when there is a massive overgrowth of multiple different types of bacteria in the vagina. With BV, there is little inflammation, so the condition is really a disturbance of the balance within the vagina rather than a true infection. In the past, the condition was called Gardnerella after the bacteria that were thought to cause it. However, the newer name, BV, reflects the fact that many species of bacteria may contribute to the overgrowth. When these multiple species of bacteria become imbalanced, the result is often a thin, grayish-white vaginal discharge with a fishy odor, both of which are often more noticeable after sex. The risk of developing BV increases if you have multiple sexual partners or a new sexual partner, if you douche, or if you smoke cigarettes (another reason to quit smoking!).

Diagnosis. The diagnosis of BV is made with three simple tests. The first is an examination of the discharge under a microscope. If you have BV, the normally smooth cells of your vagina will be coated with bacteria; these are called clue cells. In addition, the pH of your discharge will be higher (less acidic); it will go from the usual 4.0 to 5.5. The third test is called a whiff test. Your doctor will add a basic solution of potassium hydroxide to the discharge; if there is BV, this will give off a "fishy" odor. Lastly, a culture can be sent to confirm the diagnosis. Typically the culture will grow a mixture of "gram-negative anaerobes," and there will be an absence of lactobacilli.

Treatment. Treatment for BV consists of antibiotics, most commonly metronidazole taken either orally (Flagyl) or vaginally (MetroGel). Also available is the vaginal clindamycin cream (Cleocin). Oral metronidazole can cause some minor but unpleasant side effects such as nausea and a metallic taste, but it is believed to be the most effective treatment. The gels typically don't cause any side effects, although they can trigger a yeast infection.

Tinidazole (Tindamax) is a newer antibiotic that appears to have fewer side effects than metronidazole. Even if your first infection is successfully treated, recurrence is common, with more than half of all women with BV experiencing another infection within a year. Recurrent bouts may require vaginal metronidazole twice weekly for six months.

Desquamative Inflammatory Vaginitis

Desquamative inflammatory vaginitis (DIV) is a fairly rare condition in the spectrum of different causes of vaginitis. It's also poorly understood, with very few studies published on its symptoms, diagnosis, and treatment. In fact, it may not even be an infection. In other words, we're still learning.

DIV can resemble atrophic vaginitis, or thinning of the vaginal tissue, common in postmenopausal women. However, it can also occur in women with normal estrogen levels. By the time women are diagnosed, their symptoms frequently have lasted for years, and they have typically been treated dozens of times for a "vaginal infection" without long-term improvement in their symptoms.

Diagnosis. The classic symptoms of DIV are excessive yellow discharge that is very sticky and dries on the vulva like glue. The discharge is typically not foul smelling. The parts of the vulva where discharge dries become red, inflamed, and itchy. Women frequently resort to wearing panty liners all the time because the discharge ruins their underwear. In addition, DIV typically causes vestibular inflammation and dyspareunia.

The diagnosis of DIV is made when a physician examines the discharge under a microscope and sees a huge amount of white blood cells and immature vaginal cells called parabasal cells. The pH of the discharge is typically 5.5 or greater, and vaginal cultures typically show an increase in staph or strep bacteria and an absence of the "good" lactobacilli.

We're not sure what causes DIV. There are three current theories. Some vaginal infectious disease experts think that DIV may be related to an infection of an unknown organism. Another theory holds that it is due to estrogen deficiency. Lastly, some vulvar specialists think that it may be an early form of a skin disease called erosive lichen planus (see Chapter 10).

Treatment. Treatment for DIV consists of either antibiotic or corticosteroid therapy. The antibiotics most used are clindamycin (Cleocin) and metronidazole (MetroGel) in the form of either suppositories or cream inserted into the vagina every night for about two weeks.[15] Another option is to use intravaginal hydrocortisone, alone or in combination with clindamycin.[16] I (Andrew) typically treat women with a combination of clindamycin, hydrocortisone, and estrogen in a compounded cream. While this is a "shotgun" approach, it is my experience that this combination treats DIV much better than each individual medication alone or even a combination of just two of the three medications.

BOTTOM LINE

As you can see from this chapter, numerous infections can contribute to your sexual pain. Many have overlapping signs and symptoms. It is important that during any evaluation for sexual pain, your doctor conduct a thorough assessment for vaginitis and sexually transmitted infections, using all available laboratory tests to identify bacterial, viral, or fungal infections, not just a physical examination.

CHAPTER 8

Getting on Your Nerves
PUDENDAL NEURALGIA

> I'm lying on the couch cringing with pain. Maybe it's because I planted a couple of flowers or took a load of clothes out of the dryer? Things that normal people do, they all just hurt. Picking up things from the floor, bending over to tie my shoes, lifting my legs to shave them, giving the dog fresh food or water . . . even these little, everyday things hurt. I would love to pick up my grandkids or rock them to sleep at night. But with the pain I feel when I sit, that is out of the question. And we won't even mention the pain that sex would bring on.
>
> —TABITHA, SIXTY-FOUR

You learned in Chapter 2 about the role your nerves play in pain. Basically, if we didn't have those pesky things, we wouldn't feel pain, or pleasure, or touch, or, actually, any sensation. And you know from earlier chapters in this section that nerves run amok are often behind the painful sex you feel. Well, here's another nerve-related reason for your pain: pudendal neuralgia.

The condition, also called pudendal nerve entrapment or Alcock's canal syndrome, can be devastating. The pain can affect your entire vulva, including your clitoris. In addition, it can affect the perineum (that area below the vaginal opening and above the anus) as well as your entire pelvic region, whether or not you're having sex. An online survey found that an estimated 79 percent of women with the condition are depressed, while 77 percent report dyspareunia. In addition, 91 percent report pain with sitting, 89 percent report pain in their genitals, and 93 percent report perineal pain.[1]

Symptoms differ from woman to woman, but many describe their pain as burning, deeply aching, twisting/pinching, or even knifelike. Women tell us they feel as if there is a foreign body inside their rectum or vagina, and they often have problems peeing or having a bowel movement. The symptoms aren't only internal. Marli, sixty, says that her genital area "always feels cold and numb, like it is frostbitten," while Emily, forty-one, is "completely hypersensitive to touch" in the same area.

Many women with pudendal neuralgia experience some pain relief when standing, lying down, or sitting on a toilet seat or a donut-shaped cushion. These positions take pressure off the pudendal nerve. In contrast, their pain gets worse when they sit on a regular chair because this position increases pressure on the nerve.

As with many underlying causes of dyspareunia, the effects of pudendal neuralgia don't end with painful sex. As Estelle, fifty-four, describes it, "First, pudendal neuralgia all but ruined my ability to enjoy sex. Then, slowly but surely, it began to affect every area of my life." With pudendal neuralgia, day-to-day activities like sitting for longer than a few minutes (which anyone who uses a computer has to do), vacuuming, raking leaves, or shoveling snow, even lying on one side of your body at night, can lead to unbearable pain.

PUDENDAL NEURALGIA EXPLAINED

Pudendal neuralgia typically occurs following trauma or damage to the pudendal nerve. This nerve originates from the sacrum just below the base of the spine. After it leaves the sacrum, it follows a very narrow path between ligaments, the pelvic floor muscles, and the bony ridges of the pelvis. It then separates into three branches: One goes to the clitoris, another goes to the labia and perineum, and the third goes to the anus and rectum. Unfortunately, the pudendal nerve is susceptible to injury at two points along this route. The first is where the nerve travels between the sacrospinous and sacrotuberous ligaments, and the second is where the nerve travels between the pelvic floor muscles and the ischial spine of the pelvis in an area called Alcock's canal (see Figure 8.1). One estimate suggests about 1 in 100,000 women develop the condition each year, but many doctors think the numbers are much higher.[2]

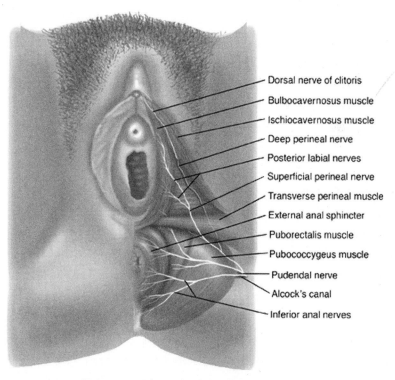

FIGURE 8.1 The path of the pudendal nerve.

The symptoms of pudendal neuralgia tend to begin gradually, although some women say their pain started all at once. The pain may occur on both sides of the pelvis or may be limited to one side; it depends on which branches are damaged. Six types of stress can harm the pudendal nerve: stretching, compression, entrapment, trauma, surgery, and inflammation. Most of the time, these triggers are no big deal. However, in women who are predisposed to pudendal neuralgia or other nerve conditions, such stresses contribute to a "cascade effect" that initiates or prolongs pain.

1. Stretch injury. Stretching a nerve to more than 15 percent of its regular length can result in permanent nerve damage. Unfortunately, the pudendal nerve can be stretched by more than 30 percent during vaginal childbirth. Stretch injuries can also result from overexercising (for example, performing deep-knee squats while holding weights).

2. Compression injury. This type of injury occurs when blood flow to the pudendal area is reduced. Compression is a particular risk during bicycle riding, especially on bikes with saddle-nose seats. I (Irwin) have studied the relationship of sexual dysfunction to bicycle riding for many years, and it is very real.

3. Traumatic injury. This type of injury occurs during an acute, or one-time, trauma. For instance, you might fall and injure your sacroiliac joint, located just above your hips next to the pudendal nerve. Snowboarders and inline skaters often fall on their buttocks, resulting in trauma to the pudendal nerve. More serious injuries, such as a fractured pelvis from a motor vehicle accident, can lead to even more severe pudendal nerve injury.

4. Entrapment. As mentioned above, the pudendal nerve travels in a very narrow pathway. The nerve can become trapped along this pathway if the sacrospinous or sacrotuberous ligaments get

thickened. In addition, the nerve can become trapped in Alcock's canal if the pelvic floor muscles become overly tight. A recent study by Stacey Futterman, a pelvic floor physical therapist, found that a tear in the hip joint can lead to pudendal nerve entrapment because the pelvic floor muscles tighten to stabilize the hip.

5. Surgeries. Hysterectomy and other surgeries involving the reproductive organs, such as laparoscopic surgery for endometriosis and vaginal prolapse, can cause nerve injury and pudendal neuralgia.

6. Inflammation. Infections that affect nerves, such as herpes or Lyme disease, can lead to inflammation of the pudendal nerve and chronic nerve pain.

SUFFERING IN SILENCE

Many women with pudendal neuralgia suffer in silence. "It took two years of steadily worsening symptoms before I decided I *had* to go to a doctor," says Cathy, sixty-four. "What finally motivated me was realizing that I had to either take early retirement or figure out what was wrong."

For many women, the presence of daily pain, the loss of a healthy sex life, and the possible loss of a job and income can be overwhelming. For these women, the choice often comes down to sitting and doing their job—and triggering chronic pain—or having an awkward, embarrassing conversation with their bosses about why they can no longer work or need extensive time off.

For women who experience pain whether sitting or standing, the condition can become completely disabling. It can be so bad, in fact, that some women contemplate suicide. "It was just one thing after another," recalls Karin, thirty-nine. "I didn't want to have sex until I felt better, but I couldn't find anything to help me feel better. My husband thought I wasn't trying hard enough. That wasn't true. I was trying so hard. Also, I still had two small children to look after. One day I just lost my motivation—that was that. I wasn't going to get out of bed or pull myself together for anything."

DIAGNOSING PUDENDAL NEURALGIA

The path to getting an accurate pudendal neuralgia diagnosis can be challenging. Amelia, forty-seven, was referred to a gynecologist, gastroenterologist, pain specialist, and psychologist before she finally found me (Andrew). The thing is, most doctors have never heard of the condition. So, many of our patients learn about their condition online or by talking with someone else in pain. Amelia finally learned what might be causing her pain when she visited a chiropractor for a completely separate injury and told him about her pelvic pain. "My chiropractor was the first person who mentioned the phrase 'pudendal nerve' in association with my pain's location. When I went home to research it, I found 'pudendal neuralgia' online and realized, that's it! That's what I have. I haven't been imagining things!"

Unfortunately, even the severe pain many women feel isn't enough to convince some doctors that they have a true, physical problem. Many health-care professionals still dismiss pudendal neuralgia as a "wastebasket" or "trash can" diagnosis—one handed out before a true diagnosis can be reached, to appease a patient, or when there's no diagnostic test for the condition. However, diagnostic tests for pudendal neuralgia do exist. The key is finding the right doctor. Your best shot at finding someone who can correctly diagnose you is to see a gynecologist, urologist, neurologist, or diagnostic specialist (think Greg House of the television program *House*).

Your doctor should perform or order the following tests:

- Physical exam. During a digital vaginal exam, the pudendal nerve can be felt at Alcock's canal. If the nerve is gently tapped with the examining finger, it may cause a pins and needles sensation (or worse pain) on the perineum, kind of like when you hit your funny bone. This is called a positive Tinel's sign and is highly suggestive of pudendal neuralgia.
- Quantitative sensory test. This noninvasive procedure uses temperature variations and vibrations to identify changes to the pudendal nerve structure or nerve fiber damage. A physician or trained technician administers this test, which should take about fifteen minutes. No needles or electric current are used, and the stimulation applied is brief, so it doesn't hurt.
- Pudendal nerve motor latency test. This test must be conducted in a neurology office by a trained technician. During the exam, the technician inserts a gloved finger into the rectum or vagina. The glove has an electrode on the tip that sends a weak electrical current through the pudendal nerve. The speed at which the nerve conducts the stimulus is recorded by a small needle inserted in the perineum. If the nerve responds more slowly than normal, it could be entrapped or damaged.
- Electromyography. This test attempts to identify any loss of nerve conduction by evaluating the electrical activity produced by your urethral and sphincter muscles (which are connected to the pudendal nerve). The neurologist inserts a two-needle or fine wire electrode into the muscle being tested and then records the levels of activity of the muscle. Women describe the procedure as slightly uncomfortable to somewhat painful, and the tested area may be sore for one or two days afterward.
- Pudendal nerve block. Typically used to treat pudendal neuralgia, this technique can also be used as a diagnostic tool. The

doctor administers an anesthetic directly into a tender segment of the pudendal nerve. I (Andrew) often perform this procedure in my office by inserting a needle through the vagina at the ischial spine, which can be seen in Figure 8.1 (it is much less painful than it sounds!). I (Irwin) insert the needle through the vestibule along the outside of the vagina to reach the ischial spine. Pudendal nerve blocks can also be performed by inserting a needle through the buttocks (my patients usually find this more painful). If your pain disappears with the nerve block, then you know you have pudendal neuralgia. For some women, a series of four to six pudendal nerve blocks with an anesthetic and steroid can provide long-term pain relief.

TREATING PUDENDAL NEURALGIA

After diagnosis, of course, comes treatment. As with many conditions underlying painful sex, there is no one-size-fits-all approach to treating pudendal neuralgia. You and your doctor will need to find the approaches that work best for you based on your symptoms, anatomy, and the initial trigger for the injury. Among the options are the following:

- Lifestyle changes. You need to make some changes in your life to prevent flare-ups. These include some you've probably already made, like doing less sitting and more standing. You should also give up (if you haven't already) activities like bicycling unless you replace your bike seat (also known as a saddle) with one that has a groove running down the center (it looks a bit like the split running through a coffee bean). Many women find that sitting on a donut-shaped cushion with an opening in the center (similar to those recommended for hemorrhoid sufferers) can help. You can find these in drugstores and medical supply stores. A small toilet trainer seat, typically used to potty-train toddlers, may also work. Other women find relief by adjusting their chairs forward or backward so that they sit on their thighs rather than the nerve. It can also help if you identify when your pain is worst and limit your activities during that time of day.

- Physical therapy. As with most conditions that underlie dyspareunia, physical therapy is a part of the treatment (see Chapter 13 for more on this). The therapist may also use hands-on techniques in your vaginal and rectal areas to try to reduce nerve constriction and/or lengthen the pelvic floor. This is important because most women with pudendal neuralgia have a very tight, short pelvic floor.

- Medical treatments. Medical treatments include the pudendal nerve blocks we discussed above, Botox injections to relax the pelvic floor muscles, and many of the medications discussed in other chapters for neuralgic pain. These include antidepressants such as Cymbalta (duloxetine), low-dose tricyclic antidepressants, and anticonvulsants like Neurontin (gabapentin).

- Alternative treatments. Some women report pain relief with alternative approaches like acupuncture, chiropractic, and rolfing (a system of deep-tissue massage designed to release misaligned muscles).

- Surgery. About one-third of women with pudendal neuralgia require surgery to reduce the nerve compression. Typically, the doctor cuts the sacrospinous or sacrotuberous ligaments to relieve the pressure on the nerve. This surgery used to be performed through large incisions in the buttocks, but today new surgical techniques allow for a less-invasive transvaginal (through the vagina) or laparoscopic approach.

BOTTOM LINE

If you suspect that you have pudendal neuralgia, don't give up! There are physicians out there who will believe you, work with you to understand your condition, and help you find relief. As with all the conditions described in this book, you can find relief from your pain.

FINDING SUPPORT

A chronic, painful condition that no one believes you have, like pudendal neuralgia, cries out for support groups. Luckily, you can find other women dealing with the same issues—along with clinical information about your condition—with just a few mouse clicks. For more information, visit the Society for Pudendal Neuralgia (http://spuninfo.org) and the Health Organization for Pudendal Education (www.pudendal.info). To talk online with other women with this problem, you can join the genital pain forum of the Institute for Sexual Medicine (http://sexualmed.org).

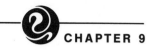

CHAPTER 9

Chronic Pelvic Pain

A SYMPTOM IN SEARCH OF A CAUSE

I began experiencing pelvic pain about three years ago. I was having urinary tract infection–like symptoms, but all the cultures were negative. At first, I suffered from aching pain in my bladder and burning pain in my urethra, which got worse during and just after urination. I found that the pain usually followed sex, so I assumed I had developed urinary tract infections as I had in my last relationship, which always went away after taking antibiotics. This time, antibiotics did not help, and my pain persisted for weeks at a time, so I decided to see a urogynecologist.

He said that I had pelvic floor muscle pain and prescribed physical therapy and Neurontin to calm the nerve pain. At this point, the pain was spreading to my entire vulva and radiated down my legs. To further explore possible causes, he performed a cystoscopy without anesthesia, and the pain was unbearable. Discouraged by my experience with this doctor, I saw four other doctors and stuck with one, who determined that I had interstitial cystitis (also known as painful bladder syndrome) and also labeled it as a chronic pelvic pain disorder.

—KATE, TWENTY-EIGHT

Many women we see describe to us a "deep" pain that gets worse during or after sex but never completely goes away. We know that this pain is not caused by the more apparent causes of dyspareunia like lichen sclerosus or chronic yeast infections because these women generally don't have pain when you touch their vulva or vagina, although they have pain with intercourse. Nonetheless, their pain is very real.

These women have chronic pelvic pain (CPP). Women with CPP describe their pain as "achy," "dull," "deep," and "relentless." The pain generally occurs in the pelvis, abdomen, below the belly button, or in the buttocks. Estimates are that CPP affects about 15 percent of women in the United States, interfering with their ability to work, have a normal life, and, of course, experience pain-free sex. In fact, 25 percent of women with CPP spend at least two days a month confined to their beds because of their pain, and 90 percent experience pain with sex. Women with CPP typically have a form of dyspareunia called deep dyspareunia and describe the location of the pain as occurring in response to deep penetration.

In addition, CPP can have permanent consequences because, all too often, doctors perform a hysterectomy (removal of the uterus) on these women. In fact, CPP is the reason for 10 to 12 percent of the more than 600,000 hysterectomies performed in the United States each year. Thus, if your doctor suggests a hysterectomy, be cautious and ask for the evidence that the uterus is causing your pain. This is important because CPP frequently persists after hysterectomy.[1]

DIAGNOSING CHRONIC PELVIC PAIN

Our job is to play detective and try to uncover the underlying cause of such pain. That's not an easy thing to do; one study found that more than half of all women with CPP never receive a definitive diagnosis.[2] Up to 40 percent of women who are diagnosed receive two or more diagnoses.

In this chapter, we explore some of the more common causes of CPP and deep dyspareunia, including interstitial cystitis (IC), pelvic congestion syndrome, endometriosis, and irritable bowel syndrome (IBS). In Chapter 7 you can read about another cause: pelvic inflammatory disease resulting from a sexually transmitted infection. Finally, in Chapter 13 we discuss pelvic floor dysfunction, which can both accompany and cause CPP.

The sections below discuss how each condition is diagnosed. But if your doctor has no clue as to what's causing your pain, he or she should do a thorough physical and pelvic examination and workup, including blood and hormone-level tests, urinalysis, pelvic ultrasound, and vaginal swabs for sexually transmitted infections. (Don't be offended! As Chapter 7 shows, it's quite possible to have an infection and not know it.) Chapter 3 covers the components of this exam and the different tests in more depth.

As emphasized in earlier chapters, it is important to be very clear and specific with your doctor about your pain. How does it feel? When does it occur? What are you doing when it occurs? Is it worse when you urinate, when you have a bowel movement, when you have your period, or when you're having sex or just after sex? Also tell your doctor about any foods that make your symptoms worse, and share your sexual history.

It is also important that you share with your doctor any history of sexual assault or sexual abuse, since both are linked to a much higher risk of CPP and certain conditions that cause pelvic pain. You can read more about the role played by sexual abuse and assault in dyspareunia in Chapter 11.

INTERSTITIAL CYSTITIS/
PAINFUL BLADDER SYNDROME

> I thought it was normal to go the bathroom every fifteen minutes, sometimes as often as twenty or thirty times a day. Until the pain began. Sometimes it was so bad I had to crawl on the floor to get to the bathroom. It felt like unending cramps, as if a heavy bowling ball were resting on top of my pelvis. Sex was out of the question; every time we made love, it hurt for days afterwards. After being continually misdiagnosed with urinary tract, bladder and kidney infections, I finally found a urologist who gave me the right diagnosis—interstitial cystitis—and began treatment.
>
> —ASHLEY, TWENTY-SIX

Interstitial cystitis, or painful bladder syndrome, is an incredibly painful condition in which you feel like you have to urinate all the time, but nothing obvious, like an infection, is wrong. The pain is chronic in both the pelvic and pubic areas. Unfortunately, it is difficult to diagnose IC, which is why so many women go undiagnosed for years. Many wind up with unnecessary hysterectomies and other surgeries in an attempt to relieve the pain.[3]

We don't know what causes IC, although some women report that their pain began after pelvic surgery or a severe bladder infection. In fact, the leading theory as to the cause of IC has to do with damage to the bladder lining. The damaged lining allows irritating components in urine to reach the underlying layer of cells, triggering pain and other symptoms.[4] At the same time, the pain and damage elicit an immune system response involving the release of inflammatory chemicals. There is also evidence that this inflammation can then cause an overgrowth of pain-transmitting nerve fibers in the bladder wall.

Sound familiar? It should since this also occurs in neuroproliferative vestibulodynia, discussed in Chapter 6. The inflammation,
coupled with the increased number of nerves, leads not only to
the pain "windup" phenomenon described in Chapter 2 but also
to pain in other nearby organs as those neurons "talk" to one another, spreading the pain message. That's why women with IC often develop vulvodynia and vice versa.

Surveys suggest that anywhere from 13 to 87 percent of women
with IC experience painful sex, with one study finding that four
out of ten women said they'd had pain during sex since they were
teenagers.[5] To understand why a condition associated with the
bladder would lead to painful sex, consider the anatomy. As you
can see in Figure 9.1, the urethra and bladder sit on top of the
vagina, cervix, and part of the uterus. So, during intercourse, these
organs may be pushed up against the bladder. That's why you often

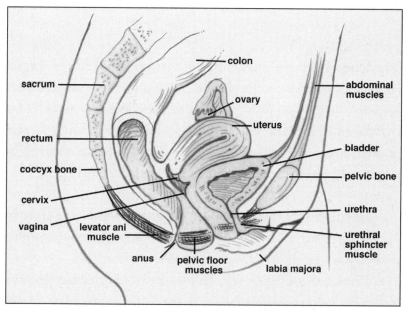

FIGURE 9.1 Female urogenital system (midsagittal section)

have to pee after sex and why frequent or deep sex can lead to bladder infections. In most women, this movement doesn't cause any discomfort. In women with IC, it can cause excruciating pain.

Another cause of sexual pain in women with IC relates to pelvic floor muscle dysfunction. Often, women have been tightening and straining these muscles for months or years as a result of the pain from the IC. Then, during sex, those muscles tighten or spasm, leading to pain.

> I have recently been diagnosed with interstitial cystitis after five years of severe bladder pain and discomfort. The bladder pain is so intense after sex, I sometimes cry for hours and can feel my pulse in my bladder. My gynecologist and urologist only told me to urinate before and after sex, which I have been doing for years to no avail. I often pass blood in my urine after sex, and the pain always follows intercourse. Is there anything else that can be done?
> —CAITLYN, TWENTY-FOUR

Diagnosis. During a physical examination, your doctor should check your pelvic floor and levator ani muscles (the muscles that hold up your pelvis). Your doctor should also culture your urine for signs of infection and check for any blood in the urine, which could be a sign of bladder cancer. Your doctor may use a variety of methods to diagnose your IC, including the following:

- Pelvic Pain and Urgency/Frequency questionnaire. A high score on this simple questionnaire (available at http://drlowellparsons .org/wst_page2.html), means you likely have IC.
- Potassium instillation test. This involves filling the bladder with a diluted potassium solution to see if it reproduces your pain,

burning, urgency, or discomfort. If you experience discomfort, the potassium solution is drained from your bladder and a "rescue solution" containing an anesthetic and steroid is put into the bladder to stop the pain and reduce inflammation.

- Cystoscopy. This test lets your doctor examine the inside of your bladder and urethra using a thin, lighted instrument called a cystoscope. The procedure is conducted under either general anesthesia, in which you are put to sleep; local anesthesia, in which an anesthetic solution or jelly is inserted into your urethra; or spinal anesthesia, which is inserted into the spinal canal. A cystoscopy enables your doctor to see if you have any ulcers on the bladder wall, called Hunner's ulcers, which may occur with IC. If you do, the doctor can take a tiny sample of the tissue for a biopsy and photograph any abnormal findings.

Sometimes the doctor fills the bladder with saline at a relatively high pressure to expand the bladder like a balloon. Patients with IC typically develop small bleeding points under the bladder surface called glomerulations after urinating out the saline. However, the process, called hydrodistensation, not only helps to diagnose IC but can provide pain relief for several months.

Finally, the doctor can also insert medications through the cystoscope to treat IC, such as anesthetics to relieve pain, steroids to reduce inflammation, and a medication that can create a new mucus barrier in the bladder (more on these treatments later in the chapter).

Treatment. Treatment for dyspareunia related to IC uses a two-pronged approach: treating the IC and then treating the pelvic floor muscle dysfunction. Both, as you probably know by now, may take months before the pain improves. So, be patient.

Medication. The only medical treatment approved specifically for IC and bladder pain is pentosanpolysulfate (Elmiron). It is thought to work by increasing the mucous layer that lines the bladder and protects the bladder wall from irritation. It is a mild blood thinner, however, so tell your doctor if you're taking any other blood thinners or are prone to bruising or heavy periods. The most common side effects are rectal bleeding, diarrhea, nausea, and, in some situations, hair loss (the hair grows back once you stop taking the drug). Be patient; it may take up to six months before you feel any significant improvement.

Other drugs used to treat IC include antihistamines to quell that overactive immune response, antidepressants such as amitriptyline (Elavil) and duloxetine (Cymbalta), and anticonvulsants such as gabapentin (Neurontin) and pregabalin (Lyrica), all of which calm the nerve endings. A procedure called bladder instillation can also help. It involves inserting a catheter into the bladder to infuse a chemical cocktail containing anesthetics such as bupivacaine or lidocaine, steroids or another anti-inflammatory medication called DMSO, and Elmiron. You hold the solution in the bladder for fifteen to thirty minutes before urinating.

Lifestyle changes. In addition to medical treatments, you need to address some lifestyle issues. Numerous foods have been linked to IC flares, including those containing caffeine or alcohol, spicy foods, and acidic foods such as tomatoes. Stress can also trigger attacks, so some relaxation training can be an important part of your treatment plan. Another approach often used is bladder training, in which you learn to wait longer and longer periods before urinating. Transcutaneous electrical nerve stimulation, which involves sending electrical pulses to the bladder area, may also help.

The second part of the treatment plan involves addressing the pelvic floor dysfunction. This can include physical therapy and myofascial release (both described in Chapter 13), internal massage, and overall strengthening and stretching of the pelvic floor muscles. Some women find relief from pain related to the pelvic floor with muscle relaxers such as intravaginal diazepam (Valium) suppositories.

PELVIC CONGESTION SYNDROME

If you feel your pain as a "chronic, dull, deep, dragging pain" in your pelvic area accompanied by heaviness and pressure, you may have pelvic congestion syndrome. This condition is caused when blood in the veins that drain the ovaries backs up, abnormally dilating the vessels and resulting in the congestion that gives the condition its name. Another way to think of it is varicose veins in your pelvis.

We don't know what causes the changes in the veins, but the condition may be related to hormones, particularly high estrogen, which we know can weaken vein walls. Additionally, changes in the veins may be related to pregnancy because there is a 60 percent increase in blood volume during pregnancy. The increased blood volume distends veins, sometimes damaging the valves that prevent the blood from backing up. This is why hemorrhoids, which are just varicose veins in the anus, are so common during and after pregnancy.

Women with pelvic congestion syndrome also tend to have thicker uterine linings and larger uteruses than women without,[6] as well as to have more menstrual problems and ovarian cysts. Other potential causes include anatomical abnormalities such as an artery crushing a vein (called nutcracker phenomena) or other cardiovascular abnormalities. A history of varicose veins, multiple pregnancies, pelvic surgery, and a "tipped" uterus all seem to increase the risk for the condition.[7]

In addition to the achiness and pain, both of which get worse when the sufferer is standing, other symptoms include a swollen vulva, increased normal vaginal discharge, backache, the need to

pee more often than normal, and varicose veins in the vulva, buttocks, or legs. Women also tend to have heavy, painful periods. And,
of course, there is the sexual pain. About 70 percent of women with
pelvic congestion have dyspareunia, and 65 percent experience pain
just after sex.

Diagnosis. Pelvic congestion often goes undiagnosed because
doctors don't know about it or don't know how to diagnose it. It
can only be diagnosed by "looking" at the veins. This can be done
with ultrasound, CT scan, or MRI.[8]

Treatment. Once the condition is diagnosed, the best treatment
for pelvic congestion is ovarian vein embolization. This procedure
is performed by an interventional radiologist (a radiologist who
also does procedures). It involves threading a catheter through the
groin to the ovarian veins and inserting tiny steel coils or ab-
sorbable sponges into the vein. This causes a clot, preventing
blood from backing up into the varicose ovarian veins.

ENDOMETRIOSIS

> My periods have always been painful, and the severity of the
> pain continues to get worse the older I get. I've been seeing
> doctors about this since I was eighteen years old. One told me I
> was too young to have endometriosis and ruled it out without
> doing any testing! Others just didn't believe me when I told them
> how it felt. But I don't know what other words I could have used
> to better express my pain and discomfort. Recently, I collapsed
> because of a cyst on my ovaries, and a laparoscopic procedure
> finally found the endometriosis.
>
> —BARB, THIRTY-SEVEN

If you have endometriosis, then tissue from the endometrium, which normally lines the inside of the uterus, is growing outside it. The endometrium thickens during the month to prepare a safe place for a fertilized egg to implant and grow. If you don't get pregnant, it breaks down and bleeds (i.e., you get your period).

With endometriosis, however, the misplaced endometrial tissue behaves just like the normal endometrium—thickening, breaking down, and bleeding—but outside of its normal habitat. These "endometriotic implants," as they're called, typically occur in the pelvic cavity and on the ovaries, tubes, and uterus. They can also affect your gastrointestinal and urinary tracts and appear in your lower abdomen. The lesions cause irritation and inflammation that can, in turn, trigger pelvic pain, painful periods, adhesions, and painful intercourse. Up to 79 percent of women with endometriosis report deep dyspareunia. The painful sex, in turn, leads to an overall negative attitude and anxiety about sex, low levels of desire, difficulty with arousal, and fewer orgasms.[9]

We still don't quite understand how endometrial tissue ends up outside of the uterus. One theory is that endometrial cells travel outside the uterus when menstrual blood flows backwards into the fallopian tubes (called retrograde or backward menstruation). Nearly all women experience some of this backward flow, however, so that doesn't explain why only some women develop endometriosis. Adolescents with obstructive reproductive tract malformations, such as a blocked or partially blocked hymen, and women with cervical stenosis, a blockage of the cervical canal, have higher rates of endometriosis, possibly because these conditions can cause higher rates of retrograde menstruation.

Other possible contributors to endometriosis include immune system defects, genetic predisposition, and the potential that some abdominal cells can transform into endometrial cells. More recently, studies have linked environmental pollutants such as PCBs and dioxin to an increased risk for endometriosis.[10]

Diagnosis. As with IC, there is no easy test to determine whether you have endometriosis. Your doctor needs to conduct a thorough medical history and exam to rule out any other medical causes for your symptoms. As with IC, make sure you provide as many specifics about your pain as possible, including what it feels like, when it's most intense, whether it's gotten worse over time, and whether it gets worse at different times during your menstrual cycle.

A physical examination can determine where the tenderness exists and locate larger abnormalities such as an endometrioma, an ovarian cyst caused by endometriosis. In addition, a physical exam in which the doctor simultaneously inserts a finger into your rectum and vagina (called a rectovaginal exam) can locate nodules in the space between the vagina and rectum that typically occur with endometriosis. Women with dyspareunia during deep-thrusting intercourse due to endometriosis may have tenderness of the cervix. In addition, the uterus may be scarred into a "tipped-back" position. An MRI can also show scarring typical of endometriosis, as well as signs of adenomyosis (endometriosis growing in the muscle fibers of the uterus).

The only way to absolutely confirm a diagnosis of endometriosis, however, is with a laparoscopy, in which the doctor inserts a thin, lighted tube with a camera on the end through your vagina or belly button to take a sample of an endometriotic implant for biopsy. It's important to get the biopsy and not just to rely on what the doctor sees during the laparoscopy because endometriosis lesions can have many different appearances, from the classic powder-burn lesions (black, brown, or gray) to atypical lesions that can be clear, red, yellow, or white. Also, other types of lesions, such as blood clots, old sutures, ovarian cancer, and even normal peritoneum, can resemble endometriotic lesions.

Whenever possible, opt for a laparoscopic over an open abdominal surgery. Not only does the camera at the end of the laparoscope allow better visualization of the lesions, but laparoscopy results in fewer adhesions, faster recovery, very little external scarring, and the ability to remove scar tissue and endometriotic implants (see below).

Treatment. Endometriosis is treated with medication, surgery, or both. Determining the best option depends on the location and severity of the lesions, your symptoms, and any other existing pelvic issues. It's also important to consider your age, reproductive plans, and duration of pain when making decisions about treatment.

Medications. Most medications for endometriosis work by reducing your body's production of estrogen. Remember, the rise and fall of your hormones—primarily estrogen and progesterone—during your menstrual cycle causes the endometrium and the endometrial implants to thicken, break down, and bleed, generating the irritation and pain. Using medication to control this ebb and flow can provide some relief. Medications used include the following:

- Danazol (Danocrine). This medication is a form of testosterone. It stops your period by reducing estrogen levels. While it was the first medication approved to treat endometriosis, it's not used that often today because of numerous side effects, including acne, swelling, weight gain, hair growth, and hot flashes. Side effects aside, one early study found that around 75 percent of women taking Danocrine said the pelvic pain and painful periods diminished, while about 60 percent said their dyspareunia improved.[11]
- Gonadotropin-releasing hormone (GnRH) agonists. These drugs, which include the nasal spray nafarelin (Synarel) and the injectable drugs leuprolide (Lupron) and goserelin (Zoladex), work by blocking production of the ovarian-stimulating luteinizing

hormone and follicle stimulating hormone. This, in turn, reduces estrogen production from the ovaries, putting you into a temporary, artificial menopause. While studies find that GnRH agonists work as well as Danazol, they also have some potentially serious side effects, including hot flashes, vaginal dryness, reduced libido, mood swings, and decreased bone density. However, you can take other medications with GnRH agonists to reduce and control many of the side effects without lowering their effectiveness.[12]

- Combination oral contraceptives. Birth control pills that contain a low dose of synthetic estrogen and progestin are often used to treat the pelvic pain associated with endometriosis. These drugs prevent ovulation and decrease menstrual flow, thus preventing the growth of those endometriotic lesions. But every woman responds differently to the hormones in oral contraceptives, so your doctor has to work to find the right type and best dosage for you. In other words, if the first trial of birth control pills doesn't work, don't give up. Some women find relief while taking the pill on the regular three weeks on, one week off schedule; others find that taking the pill continuously for three to four months before taking a break for a light period works better.

  While birth control pills can work well, studies find that GnRH agonists do a better job at relieving painful periods and dyspareunia.[13] Side effects of oral contraceptives may include nausea, headache, abnormal uterine bleeding, and blood clots, particularly in women over thirty-five who smoke, as well as decreased sexual function.

Surgical options. Medications aren't a cure for endometriosis. GnRH agonists and Danazol can only be taken for a few months. Once you stop taking them, symptoms eventually return. That's where laparoscopy comes in. If you undergo the procedure for diagnosis, and your doctor finds lesions, he or she can remove them at the same time. One study found that six months after the procedure, women reported a 62 percent improvement in their pain compared to a 24 percent reduction in the control group.[14] In a similar study, 80 percent of women reported relief from their symptoms after undergoing laparoscopy to remove their endometrial lesions, compared to 32 percent of women who had the procedure for diagnostic purposes (without removing the lesions).[15]

Presacral and uterosacral neurectomy are sometimes performed along with laparoscopy. These surgical procedures cut the nerves that transmit pain from the uterus. This can work to relieve some of the pelvic pain but won't affect lesions located far from the uterus. Together with laparoscopic removal of visible lesions, studies find these procedures can reduce painful periods and chronic pelvic pain and improve dyspareunia more than removing the lesions alone.[16]

If you're finished having children and your pain is severe, you might want to consider a hysterectomy and oophorectomy (removal of your ovaries). Removing the ovaries, which produce most of your body's estrogen, slashes estrogen levels and ends menstruation. Although removing the ovaries is somewhat controversial, one study found that endometriosis recurred in 60 percent of women who had a hysterectomy but retained one or both ovaries, as opposed to in only 10 percent of women who had both ovaries removed.[17]

IRRITABLE BOWEL SYNDROME

As if the IBS wasn't bad enough on its own, now I find that my symptoms get worse the day after I've had sex. I get terrible pain and diarrhea. Today there is a constant throbbing in my bowels and very bad gas. And it's not like I'm having sex that often; the deep pain of the IBS makes that the last thing on my mind.

—MEGAN, FORTY

Irritable bowel syndrome is not actually a disease but, rather, a collection of symptoms that can't be explained by any injury or known disease, hence the word "syndrome." Key symptoms include chronic pain, usually in the lower abdomen, as well as constipation, diarrhea, or both (mixed). An estimated 10 to 20 percent of the population is thought to have IBS, and 60 to 70 percent of that group are women.[18] In fact, if gynecologists knew more about IBS and were more diligent in considering it as a potential diagnosis in women with chronic pelvic pain, many women could avoid the numerous tests and procedures they undergo and receive treatment—and relief—much sooner.[19]

We don't know what causes IBS, but we think that it relates to the connection between the brain in your head and the "brain" in your gut, called the brain-gut axis.[20] The system relies on a complex interplay between neurotransmitters and the immune system. Stress or any significant change to the stomach, colon, or bowel can disrupt that delicate balance. For instance, symptoms often seem to start after a bad case of gastroenteritis (i.e., stomach flu or food poisoning), an inflammatory infection, or even abdominal or pelvic surgery. In one study, 17 percent of women who underwent elective gynecological surgery developed abdominal pain three to twelve months after surgery.[21]

With those neurotransmitter signals out of whack, people with IBS don't process signals from the gut correctly, leading to a lower threshold for pain and a greater awareness of any painful sensations in their gut. If this sounds familiar, it should. Both symptoms are also seen in women with PVD, although the enhanced pain and attention to sensations come from the vulvar region, not the gut.[22]

Studies find that up to 78 percent of women with IBS also report dyspareunia,[23] while between 29 and 79 percent of women with chronic pelvic pain also have IBS.[24] Women with IBS also report lower libidos, greater sexual pain, and more severe IBS symptoms after having sex. No wonder they try to avoid intercourse![25] We also find that women with IBS and sexual problems are more likely to have a history of sexual abuse or pelvic floor dysfunction (for more on sexual abuse and dyspareunia, see Chapter 11).

Diagnosis. As with similar conditions, it's quite likely that you will see more than one doctor before getting a diagnosis of IBS. Once diagnosed, make sure you feel good about your doctor and that you work well as a team. There's evidence that people with IBS who have a good relationship with their doctor have fewer follow-up visits, suggesting that they benefit more from treatment.[26]

Irritable bowel syndrome used to be a diagnosis of exclusion, meaning that if your doctor couldn't find any other reason for your symptoms, he or she diagnosed you with IBS. Today, however, there are specific guidelines for diagnosing IBS without subjecting people to painful, invasive, and expensive tests. For instance, the guidelines don't recommend a colonoscopy in people under fifty whose symptoms suggest IBS. Instead, the criteria call for a diagnosis if you have had recurrent abdominal pain or discomfort at least three days a month in the last three months with two or more of the following characteristics[27]:

- The pain improves when you have a bowel movement.
- The pain begins when the frequency of your bowel movements changes (they become more or less frequent).
- The pain begins with a change in the form or appearance of your stool.

If you have the diarrheal or mixed form of IBS, your doctor should also test you for celiac sprue, an autoimmune disease in which gluten and other proteins found in grains like wheat, barley, and rye damage the lining of the small intestine.

Treatment. There is no cure for IBS, only various treatments that can help improve and manage your symptoms. All treatment should begin with understanding your condition and the fact that it is not curable.

Diet. There is no "IBS diet." Instead, you might try making several dietary changes, such as cutting out dairy products, gas-producing foods like beans, onions, and celery, fructose and other carbohydrates, and even gluten-containing foods to see if your symptoms improve. You can also experiment with increasing your fiber through diet, supplements, or both, especially if you have constipation-type IBS.

Psychosocial therapy. If your symptoms are related to stress, you might benefit from hypnosis, biofeedback, or psychotherapy to reduce your anxiety levels. Such approaches can also help you learn how to cope better with your condition, increase your tolerance to pain, and improve overall behaviors that could reduce your symptoms.[28]

Medications. Unlike with many medical conditions, medication should be used in addition to other approaches, not as the focus of treatment. Which drug your doctor prescribes depends on the type of IBS you have (i.e., diarrhea predominant or constipation predominant). Medications include the following:

- Antispasmodic agents. These drugs affect the smooth muscle of the colon, relaxing it to prevent pain-causing spasms, diarrhea, gas, and bloating. They include dicyclomine (Bentyl, among other brand names), hyoscyamine (Levbid and Anaspaz, among other brand names), mebeverine (Colofac), and pinaverine

(Pavabid). Side effects depend on the drug used. That's why it's important that you always read the package inserts that come with any medication. They list potential side effects or interactions with other medications that even your doctor may be unaware of. In addition, your pharmacist is an excellent resource for information about potential side effects and drug-drug interactions.

- Antidepressants. Antidepressants, including tricyclic antidepressants and possibly selective serotonin reuptake inhibitors, can improve the function of those neurotransmitters in the gut and brain that are implicated in IBS. An analysis of thirteen studies of 789 people with IBS found that antidepressants worked significantly better than placebo at relieving pain and other IBS symptoms one to three months after the start of treatment.[29] Tricyclic antidepressants such as amitriptyline (Elavil) and imipramine (Tofranil) can also improve diarrhea if you have that type of IBS, but they shouldn't be used if you have constipation-type IBS.

- Antidiarrheal agents. Loperamide (Imodium A-D) can help if you have diarrhea-type IBS. Possible side effects include constipation and stomach cramps.

- Selective 5-HT3 receptor antagonists. Drugs in this category include alosetron (Lotronex), which is only approved for use in women, and the antinausea drugs ondansetron (Zofran) and granisetron (Granisol). These drugs can improve bowel movements and reduce pain. They are primarily used in people with diarrhea-type IBS. Possible side effects include constipation and gastrointestinal discomfort and pain.

- Lubiprostone. This drug is approved for women with constipation-type IBS. The most common side effect is nausea. It is generally reserved for people in whom other approaches haven't worked.

BOTTOM LINE

Chronic pelvic pain is not a disease in and of itself but a condition related to some underlying physiologic process run amuck. If you're persistent, you'll find the right doctor and receive the right diagnosis and treatment. The information in this chapter should certainly help with that! Just remember that you are ultimately the one in charge of your body; you deserve respect and to have attention paid to your symptoms, no matter how diverse; and you deserve to be a partner with your health-care team in identifying and treating the underpinnings of your chronic pelvic pain.

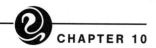

CHAPTER 10

When the Pain Is Skin Deep

About eight years ago, I began to experience severe itching in my vaginal area. I tried numerous over-the-counter remedies and also tried to diagnose myself via the Internet. I made an appointment with a gynecologist. She noticed a shiny white spot on my vulva, biopsied it, and told me I had lichen sclerosus. I guess I am one of the lucky ones who actually had a biopsy before being tested to death for other possible causes. Soon after, I began to experience narrowing of the vaginal opening and anal problems as well. I found a website for people with lichen sclerosus and joined that group, which has given me so much information.

I still have trouble controlling the lichen sclerosus and have a nonexistent sex life. It is painful to have sex and frustrating for my husband and me. He doesn't understand and has basically accused me of concocting this in my head. I've told no one about this other than my physician and my husband. It is a horrifying and embarrassing position to be in.

—FRANCES, THIRTY-FIVE

Quick: What doctor would you call if you had pain and itching in your vulva and pain with sex? A gynecologist, urologist, or dermatologist? Chances are, you didn't answer dermatologist. That's because most people think about acne, rashes, wrinkles, and skin cancer when they think about dermatologists. Yet, the underlying cause of dyspareunia for many women lies not in their nerves but in their skin. Unfortunately, just as dermatologists are not trained to perform pap smears, gynecologists are rarely trained in the variety of skin conditions that can affect the vulva and vagina. Skin conditions such as contact dermatitis, lichen sclerosus (LS), lichen planus (LP), and lichen simplex chronicus (LSC) can all result in pain during sex. The pain can range from mild to severe and disabling and may be accompanied by other symptoms such as severe itching, pain, tearing, and scarring.

Like Frances, many women are so embarrassed by the resulting changes in their vulvas and vagina that they avoid sex altogether. Their shame also keeps them from telling their health-care professional about the problem. The result? Lack of diagnosis and treatment (or the wrong treatment), continuing symptoms, and devastating effects on their lives.

That's why, as we keep stressing, it is so important that you tell your doctor about everything happening in your body, whether or not you think it's related to your pain (for a refresher on how to talk to your doctor, revisit Chapter 3). And if your gynecologist or primary care doctor does happen to notice that your pain may be related to a skin condition, ask for a referral to a dermatologist. This is particularly important since, left untreated, vulvovaginal skin conditions can become cancerous or literally destroy the vulva and parts of the vagina. However, if diagnosed early, most can be treated with topical medications. In addition to early diagnosis, accurate diagnosis is also key. Even though several of the skin conditions described here have similar names, they are distinct diseases.

YOUR IMMUNE SYSTEM AND DYSPAREUNIA

Many of the conditions described here are the result of an out-of-whack immune system. The immune system's primary role is to protect you from harmful substances—bacteria, viruses, fungi, and so forth. When immune system cells learn that some invader threatens, they move into action, unleashing a series of inflammatory proteins designed to eradicate the threat.

Your immune system is not, however, supposed to unleash that force against your own cells. Immune system cells recognize your own cells through a combination of proteins and sugars on their surface—your individual signature. Sometimes, however, this system goes awry; your immune cells stop recognizing your personal protein-and-sugar signature and attack your body's own cells, damaging them and the surrounding tissue. This is what happens in autoimmune disorders, such as lupus and rheumatoid arthritis—and, as you'll see below, lichen sclerosus and lichen planus.

In other instances, your immune system overreacts to relatively harmless proteins, such as pollen or even the chemicals that make up the scent in your new bath oil. Such hypersensitivity is behind allergies and the redness, itching, and inflammation of an allergic reaction, including the allergic contact dermatitis that often underlies dyspareunia. One reason topical or systemic steroids are prescribed so often in these conditions is that they suppress, or calm, the immune system, short-circuiting the inflammatory response responsible for your pain.

DIAGNOSIS

Most dermatologic causes of your dyspareunia are diagnosed clinically—by examining the area for any cracks, ulcers, color or texture changes, or loss of normal skin architecture. Your doctor may perform a vulvoscopy (an examination of the vulva using a microscope) and, if any abnormalities are found, perform a skin biopsy to confirm the diagnosis and to make sure there are no pre-cancerous cells.

IRRITANT AND ALLERGIC CONTACT DERMATITIS

Irritant contact dermatitis (ICD) is a skin condition marked by vulvar itching, burning, and irritation. It is one of the most common vulvar skin conditions, affecting approximately one out of four women who visit vulvar specialty clinics. The condition occurs when the relatively sensitive skin and mucosa of the vulva encounters irritating chemicals. We find the condition is more common these days because more women are using scented products in and around their vulvas, many of which contain these irritating chemicals. Even Dove soap, advertised as being "99 percent pure," contains fourteen different chemicals, any of which can cause ICD. Other products to blame for rising ICD rates include scented or treated menstrual pads, panty liners, toilet paper, fabric detergents and softeners, feminine sprays, and medications for yeast infections. Even products marketed to treat vaginal itching, such as Vagisil Feminine Cream (benzocaine), contain chemicals that can cause ICD or make it worse.

A closely related condition is allergic contact dermatitis (ACD). Here, the offending chemical not only causes irritation but activates the body's immune system, resulting in that hypersensitivity described above. The itching, redness, and pain of ACD is the result of inflammatory chemicals called histamines, which immune system cells release in response to a perceived threat that is really just a protein from the product you're using. The pain and itching of ACD are usually much worse than with ICD and are exacerbated with each exposure to the offending chemical.

Treating Irritant or Allergic Contact Dermatitis

The best way to treat both ICD and ACD is to stop using the product that's causing the problem. Since it's often difficult to tell exactly which product that is, we recommend that our patients end all chemical exposure in the vaginal/vulvar area. That means washing the area with warm water only (i.e., with no soap or liquid cleaners); using unscented, natural (undyed) toilet paper and menstrual pads; and hand-washing your underwear in hot water only and air-drying it. You may also need to apply a topical steroid to the vulva for about a month to halt the inflammation.

LICHEN SCLEROSUS

> I suffer from lichen sclerosus and can no longer enjoy intercourse. Just wiping with toilet paper tears my skin.
> —BRENDA, FIFTY-TWO

Lichen sclerosus (LS) is a chronic autoimmune inflammatory condition that usually affects the skin of the vulva and that surrounding the anus. It is a common cause of dyspareunia. Women with LS experience intense vulvar itching, burning, pain, tearing, decreased clitoral sensation, and changes to their vulvar anatomy. The condition affects about one in seventy women, with women about thirteen times more likely to develop it than men.[1] About 10 percent of patients are preadolescent girls, 40 percent are premenopausal women, and 50 percent are menopausal women. In about 10 percent of people with the condition, LS affects nonvulvar skin.

The condition occurs as white blood cells from the immune system accumulate in the vulvar skin, releasing inflammatory chemicals and leading to the chronic inflammation that is the hallmark of the disease. Over time, the vulvar skin loses its color, or pigmentation, and becomes crinkled or waxy (it has been described as looking like cigarette paper or wax paper), cracking and tearing easily. The labia may become stuck together, narrowing the opening of the vagina, which tears during penetration. The prepuce (hood) of the clitoris may scar on the top, effectively burying the clitoris under scar tissue; this is called clitoral phimosis (see below).

Unfortunately, women often suffer with such awful symptoms for years before getting diagnosed. In addition, the chronic inflammation results in cancer of the vulva in about 4 percent of women with LS. Fortunately, with proper treatment we can improve the symptoms, prevent scarring, and significantly reduce the risk of cancer.

Treating Lichen Sclerosus

Since LS is, first and foremost, the product of an overactive immune system, the goal of treatment is to suppress the immune system. We can't suppress it entirely, however, or you would have no protection at all against infection. So, we try to suppress just the immune system in the vulvar skin.

Since the early 1990s, the mainstay of LS treatment has been clobetasol (Temovate), an ultrapotent topical steroid. If used correctly, Temovate and similar steroids bring on remission within two to eight weeks. The risks include thinning of the skin, rebound reactions after stopping the steroids, stretch marks, suppression of the adrenal glands, and increased risk of fungal infections. However, with proper use, these risks are minimal (see "Dr. Andrew Goldstein's Tips for Treating Lichen Sclerosus").

Another class of drugs called topical calcineurin inhibitors, typically used to treat eczema and other skin conditions, also show promise in treating LS.[2] Pimecrolimus (Elidel) and tacrolimus

(Protopic) also suppress the immune system but without steroids. Thus, they don't carry the risk of skin thinning. However, a clinical trial that I (Andrew) recently completed comparing clobetasol to Elidel showed that clobetasol worked slightly better.[3]

You may also need to take an oral antifungal, antibiotic, or both for the first week or two of treatment because the cracks, fissures, and erosions from the inflammation leave your skin open to infection. Once the LS improves, topical estrogen and testosterone cream can help increase the moistness, elasticity, and lubrication of the vulvar skin, while surgery can correct the scarring. In time, you

DR. ANDREW GOLDSTEIN'S TIPS FOR TREATING LICHEN SCLEROSUS

- Use clobetasol ointment instead of cream. It is easier to apply and, unlike many creams, doesn't contain alcohol, which can irritate the skin.
- Use Temovate brand instead of generic clobetasol if possible. It is simply absorbed into the skin better than the generic and therefore works better. Ask your doctor to write on the prescription that Temovate should not be switched for the generic.
- Soak in warm water for fifteen minutes to soften the skin before applying the Temovate so that your skin can absorb the ointment better.
- Use a mirror to see the areas affected by LS, and use only enough of the ointment to cover the affected area, usually between a pea- and lima bean–sized amount.
- Gently rub in the ointment for two to three minutes until it is completely absorbed.
- Use the ointment daily until all evidence of LS is gone. Then slowly taper to once or twice a week for a year. Even though the package instructions say to use it for no more than two weeks, in our experience we find that two weeks is simply not enough time to improve the condition.

should be able to regain full sexual function, and your clitoris should be as sensitive (in a good way!) as ever. However, the LS isn't cured; it requires lifelong treatment to keep it in remission. Women with LS also have a higher risk for other autoimmune disorders, including thyroid disease, vitiligo (loss of skin coloring), and pernicious anemia (inability to absorb vitamin B12).

CLITORAL PHIMOSIS[4]

> My pain seems so unreal, so strange. I can have sex and can have orgasm, but afterwards I have severe pain in the area around my clitoris. It feels like intense pressure, as if someone dropped a ten-pound weight on my clitoris. It is so bad that I avoid even thinking about sex because if I get aroused, I will be in pain for days. I tried to look at my clitoris to see what the problem is, but I can't seem to find it. I know it was there in the past.
>
> —KARA, FORTY-EIGHT

Kara went to over a dozen different physicians before she came to see me (Irwin) at San Diego Sexual Medicine. A thorough exam revealed the telltale skin changes of LS. In addition, just as Kara had mentioned, her clitoris was not visible; her prepuce had completely scarred over her clitoris, leaving her with clitoral phimosis. She treated her LS with Temovate ointment, but this did not correct the clitoral phimosis; nor did it solve her pain with arousal. For this problem I performed a simple surgery to reopen the prepuce called a dorsal slit procedure. Fortunately, after a two-week recovery, Kara is once again able to have sex without pain, and since her clitoris is now free from scar tissue, she is more easily aroused.

LICHEN PLANUS[5]

> In 2003, I began experiencing pain during intercourse. I had always used tampons and had frequent intercourse with my husband with no problems. My doctor diagnosed me with lichen planus. It has caused the complete atrophy of my inner labia, and my clitoral hood is partially fused over. It is progressive and requires constant vigilance to stop its effects from taking over. The pain comes and goes—some days are great, and I don't even notice it; other days are horrible, and it's all I can think about. I have tried so many different treatments and learned that for most women treatment is comprised of several different modalities, not just one magic bullet. Now, almost six years later, because of all my research, treatment, and hard work, I am able to sometimes have intercourse without pain.
>
> —CASSANDRA, FORTY-NINE

Like LS, lichen planus (LS) is a chronic autoimmune skin disease. However, several differences between the two conditions affect diagnosis and treatment. In LS, only a small percentage of women have skin changes on nonvulvar parts of their bodies. In contrast, only one out of four women with LP has any vulvovaginal involvement; the condition is more likely to affect the mouth and gums than the vulva or vagina. Another major distinction is that LP affects both the vulva and vagina, whereas LS never goes into the vagina. Thus, LP can cause both vulvar and vaginal scarring. In addition, in LP erosions on the mucous membranes of the vulva and vagina are more common than the wax paper appearance of LS. These erosions often have lacy borders called Wickham's stria.

Treating Lichen Planus

Unfortunately, LP is often much more difficult to control than LS. Some women will have good success with ultrapotent steroids such as clobetasol and the calcineurin inhibitors (Elidel and Protopic). However, in more difficult cases, systemic steroids such as oral prednisone may be necessary. If the condition affects your vagina, it's also important that a vaginal dilator be used to prevent vaginal scarring. You use the dilator to apply the steroid to the ulcers in the vagina, which also helps prevent the vaginal walls from sticking to each other.

LICHEN SIMPLEX CHRONICUS[6]

Unlike LS, LP, and ACD, lichen simplex chronicus (LSC) is not an autoimmune disorder. Instead, LSC is caused by chronic itching and scratching. One of several initiating factors—an allergic reaction, a fungal infection, or irritation due to heat and moisture—starts the itching and scratching. Then a chain reaction occurs in which the scratching brings mast cells (a specialized type of white blood cell) to the area, where they secrete a protein called histamine that causes even more itching. The itching leads to more scratching, and the itch-scratch-itch cycle takes on a life of its own, even after the original irritant is gone. The skin responds to the chronic scratching by thickening and becoming "lichenified." The scratching, which often occurs during sleep, can be so severe that some women scratch all their hair away and create pits in the skin from gouging.

Treating Lichen Simplex Chronicus

The goal of treatment in LSC is to break the itch-scratch-itch cycle. This requires stopping all chemical exposure to the vulva (just like in irritant contact dermatitis) and treating all infections. The inflammation caused by the scratching is treated with topical steroids, while the itching can be soothed by applying ice to the vulva and taking a low-dose tricyclic antidepressant such as amitriptyline to prevent scratching at night. Once the itch-scratch-itch cycle has been broken, the topical steroid will quickly treat all remaining inflammation. Unlike LS or LP, once successfully treated, your LSC is cured and shouldn't return unless something else starts the itch-scratch-itch cycle again.

HIDRADENITIS SUPPURATIVA[7]

Hidradenitis suppurativa (HS) is a chronic inflammatory condition in which the sweat glands in the genital area become clogged. It's similar to acne. In fact, some think it might be an unusual form of acne. The trapped sweat, however, quickly becomes infected with bacteria, causing inflammation, pain, pus, and odor. The infection leads to abscesses that sometimes develop into fistulas, or holes, in the vulvar area and vagina. Stress and being overweight can make the condition worse, and there is some thought that smoking may contribute to it. There is also a genetic component, so if a parent or other close relative has had HS, you're more likely to get it. The condition is also related to high androgen levels and typically flares just before or during menstruation, improving during pregnancy.

Unfortunately, HS is one of those poorly understood conditions, making a quick diagnosis difficult and frustrating. One study of 164 women found it took an average of seven years before they were diagnosed.[8] Women with the condition typically have chronic pain, depression, a terrible sex life, and overall poor quality of life. Yet, HS can be diagnosed from the characteristic red and inflamed sweat glands. No biopsy is needed.

Treating Hidradenitis Suppurativa

If you're suffering from HS, don't shave your pubic hair as this can cause increase inflammation. Taking warm baths and wearing loose-fitting clothing can help with the pain and prevent new lesions from developing. Medical treatment typically begins with antibiotics to eradicate infection and oral contraceptives to reduce androgen levels. In women who require stronger treatment, there's some evidence that drugs that reduce androgen levels, like finasteride (Proscar, among other brands) and spironolactone (Aldactone, among other names), may help. More intensive treatment includes the use of immune-suppressing medications such as infliximab (Remicade) or etanercept (Enbrel), as well as steroids injected directly into the lesions.[9] In very serious cases, you may need surgery to remove the lesions.

BOTTOM LINE

As this chapter clearly shows, dermatologic conditions play a big role in sexual pain. Since few gynecologists or even primary care physicians are trained in dermatologic diseases that affect the genitals, if you suspect a skin condition is behind your pain, make an appointment with a board-certified dermatologist and ask if they have experience treating vulvar skin disease. And don't be embarrassed!

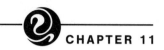

CHAPTER 11

Delving into the Past

THE ROLE OF TRAUMA AND ABUSE IN SEXUAL PAIN

> I was raped multiple times by both of my sexual partners. I also have flashbacks and for many years occluded the memories of trauma. With the tender help of my physical therapist and the intimate nature of our work together, in addition to working with a sex therapist, I have started processing the trauma and sexual abuse and have talked to my husband about my history.
>
> —DANIELLE, THIRTY-NINE

An estimated one in ten women have been forced to have sex at some point in their lives, while 20 to 25 percent of college-aged women say they experienced an attempted or completed rape while in school. Even more shameful is the fact that 60 percent of women who were raped were assaulted before age eighteen. Among adult women who have been raped, one-third experienced a physical injury resulting from their attack.[1]

We are not making up these statistics. They are publicly available on the Centers for Disease Control and Prevention's website (www.cdc.gov). They highlight a terrifying and horrendous reality:

Women in this country (and many others) face a constant threat of sexual violence.

And that violence, if it occurs, can affect them not only physically and emotionally for the rest of their lives but also sexually. One review of seven studies found that women with a history of sexual abuse were more than twice as likely to experience dyspareunia.[2] Unfortunately, most women keep their abuse to themselves. A survey of more than five hundred women in a family practice clinic found that although one in five said they'd been sexually assaulted at some point in their lives, just 2 percent had ever discussed it with a physician, and nearly half had never told anyone.[3]

We've emphasized throughout this book how important it is that you share any sexual or physical abuse history with your doctor. That's because, although the conclusion is somewhat controversial, it appears that such abuse underlies some forms of dyspareunia in some women. Why is it controversial? Well, as you'll see, the scientific support is mixed. But another reason for the controversy is the fear that if we pin the blame for the pain on abuse, we will let medicine off the hook, and doctors won't have to investigate other issues. As Corren, twenty-six, told us, "I sought help for my pain when I was twenty-three on active duty in the army and had given birth to my daughter (now three). Every doctor I went to asked me the exact same question: Did I have a history of sexual abuse? I answered yes, and they nodded and smiled knowingly, then proceeded to tell me that my mind was doing it to me."

While the mind is a powerful thing, it is not "doing" anything to you, and that notion should not lead to a minimization or discounting of your condition. The scientific reality is that we do see a link between sexual abuse and many conditions related to dyspareunia, including chronic pelvic pain, irritable bowel syndrome (IBS), and interstitial cystitis (for more on all three, see Chapter 9).[4] For instance, 40 to 58 percent of women with IBS and 49 percent of women with interstitial cystitis report they were sexually or physically abused as a child or adult—rates far higher than those found in pain-free women.[5] Studies also show that women with IBS have higher rates of sexual abuse—including threatened sex, incest, forced intercourse, lifetime sexual victimization, severe lifetime sexual trauma, and severe childhood sexual abuse—than women with similar gastrointestinal conditions.[6] However, there is little evidence that women with vulvodynia have higher rates of sexual or physical abuse than women without.[7] Also, keep in mind that not every woman who has been abused develops dyspareunia; nor does every woman with dyspareunia have a history of sexual or physical abuse.

EXPLAINING THE CONNECTIONS

In conditions in which there is a relationship between abuse and dyspareunia, however, it isn't clear whether the abuse caused the dyspareunia or the linkage is incidental (i.e., related to other factors). Just consider that women who have been sexually abused have more medical and psychological problems, including anxiety, depression, sleep disorders, pelvic pain, and breast disease, regardless of their sexual health. They are also more likely to experience psychological problems physically (i.e., to experience chronic pain when they are depressed) and to engage in risky behaviors, such as having several sexual partners and abusing alcohol and drugs.[8]

The problem is that it is very difficult to design studies and run the statistical analyses required to get at direct causes. Did the sexual abuse cause the depression, which is causing the pain? Or did the abuse lead to the pelvic pain, which then triggered the anxiety? Or were the anxiety and depression present before the abuse? That's why, in this context, we use phrases like "associated with," "relationship to," and "linkage between" rather than the word "cause."[9]

Having said that, there are some theories concerning the link-ages between sexual abuse and sexual pain:

- Recall bias. This theory holds that women who are more likely to remember abuse are also more likely to accept the idea that there is a psychological reason for their physical symptoms.
- Cognitive theory. This theory focuses on the mind, suggesting that negative thoughts and difficulties coping with stress like that from abuse may lead to problems adjusting to illness, in-creasing complaints about pain and pain-related behaviors.
- Physiologic theory. This theory holds that a traumatic incident, such as sexual assault or abuse involving the genitals, makes the nerves in that area more sensitive to pain signals. It may also be that such a negative stimulus can, over time, create a dysfunc-tional feedback loop between the pelvic muscles, the dorsal horn (the nerves that supply the pelvic/genital area), and altered parts of the brain related to pain, fear, and anxiety, like those Caroline identified with her MRI studies (see page 29 for more on this).[10] Basically, the abuse changes the pain/brain feedback loop. In fact, there is some evidence that sexual abuse does change pain signals in the brain,[11] with one study showing that women with a history of abuse and IBS had more activity in the area of the brain associated with pain and stress reactions.[12]

TREATING ABUSE-RELATED SEXUAL PAIN

We can recommend no magic formula, drug, or procedure to treat this underlying cause of dyspareunia. Instead, you will need to work closely with a good therapist to learn to process the trauma you experienced. Cognitive behavioral therapy (CBT) is one good approach (see Chapter 14); another is Eye Movement Desensitization and Reprocessing, a comprehensive, integrative psychotherapy approach that contains elements of other effective therapeutic approaches, including CBT and interpersonal (the classic "talk" therapy) methods. The goal is to help you process the past experiences that led to your current pain; understand situations that trigger dysfunctional emotions, beliefs, and sensations; and develop new behaviors to improve your mental health and, thus, your pain. One procedure used during treatment has you think about past memories and current triggers, while you focus on something outside yourself, like a statue. Eventually, you may experience new insights or associations in conjunction with the memories.

One key is finding the right therapist. Any therapist won't do. Look for one who specializes or has significant experience in working with women with a history of sexual abuse or sexual violence. And contact support groups. The "Sexual Abuse and Violence Resources" box provides several national resources that can point you toward support groups (online and in person), as well as medical, legal, and mental health resources.

SEXUAL ABUSE AND VIOLENCE RESOURCES

National Organization for Victim Assistance (NOVA)
www.trynova.org

National Sexual Violence Resource Center (NSVRC)
www.nsvrc.org

The National Alliance to End Sexual Violence Foundation (NAESV)
www.naesv.org

Institute on Violence, Abuse, and Trauma (IVAT)
www.ivatcenters.org

The National Online Resource Center on Violence Against Women (VAWnet)
www.vawnet.org

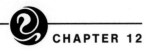

CHAPTER 12

And Baby Makes Three

THE ROLE OF CHILDBIRTH
IN SEXUAL PAIN

> Sex definitely hurt after I had my baby. Even beyond the six weeks after birth when my doctor said I could have sex again, intercourse was very painful. In addition to the pain and vaginal dryness and the fact that I'd had an episiotomy, I think my general exhaustion from sleep deprivation (I was breast-feeding at night) had a big influence. I had a very hard time keeping my interest and libido up for more than few minutes. Altogether, it took about six months after giving birth to get any pleasure from sex.
>
> —MONICA, TWENTY-EIGHT

If you've ever seen a vaginal birth, then it will come as no surprise that the trauma a woman's body experiences during childbirth can affect her sexual pleasure and cause sexual pain. About half of the 4 million women who have babies each year report pain with sex three months after delivery, and many continue to experience painful sex even a year later.[1] More than half of women who say they had little or no trauma during the delivery still report pain the first time they have sexual intercourse, and 18 percent still experience pain even after six months.[2] Childbirth can lead to painful sex regardless of the type of delivery—uncomplicated vaginal delivery with or without tearing or episiotomy, complicated vaginal delivery, or even cesarean section. Your postpartum sex life can even be affected by breast-feeding.

Painful sex, on top of the upheaval of a newborn baby and the emotional mood swings tied to the fluctuating hormones of postpartum life, can be devastating. When a patient comes to me (Irwin) in pain after childbirth, I check these very hormones to determine if they may be part of the problem. After all, the last thing you need at this point is more stress and insecurity about your body. Yet, as discussed Chapter 4, painful sex can also interfere with your relationship with your partner, who may not understand why you're not eager to resume lovemaking immediately, once the doctor gives the green light. He may already be feeling ignored and discarded, given your focus on the baby. He thought he'd at least get you back through lovemaking. Hah! Not quite.

The good news is that painful sex following childbirth is rarely permanent. It tends to improve significantly between three and six months after birth and, for most women, has returned to normal by eighteen months after childbirth.[3] However, the fact that the pain is temporary doesn't mean you have to grin and bear it or abstain from sex. If you're still pregnant and reading this, there are things you can do now to reduce the likelihood of dyspareunia later. If you've already given birth, several effective treatments can limit the pain until it dissipates on its own.

WHAT'S BEHIND THE PAIN?

I have a seven-month-old. Since her birth, I have found it difficult to have sex with my husband. I had an episiotomy, and ever since

then intercourse feels like a knife entering inside me. It has eased
a little over time but is still very painful, and, to say the least, I do
not want to have sex.

—KATE, TWENTY-SEVEN

The more traumatic the birth, the more postpartum sex is likely to
hurt. The greatest culprits, of course, are tearing in the perineum
(the area between the vagina and anus) and effects of an episiotomy (a surgical cut in the perineum to allow more room for
the baby's head). Surprisingly, there's no good evidence that one is
more likely to cause postpartum sexual pain than the other.[4] However, there is excellent evidence that routine use of episiotomy increases the risk of rectal tears and complications with healing.[5] So,
even beyond the issue of postpartum dyspareunia, we strongly dis-
courage the use of episiotomy except when the life of the baby is
in danger. Having an assisted birth—in which the doctor or midwife delivers the baby with a vacuum or forceps—also increases
the likelihood of postpartum dyspareunia because it increases the
risk of vaginal or rectal tearing or the need for episiotomy.

In rare cases, labor and delivery can damage the coccyx (tailbone)
and the surrounding soft tissue. Such damage, called coccydynia, is
characterized by constant pain that gets worse when you move or sit
down. Of course, having sex just makes it hurt even more! Finally,
there is the rare risk of pudendal nerve injury. This can occur during
the final phase of labor when your legs are pulled back toward your
head as you try to push the baby out. The position itself stretches the
pudendal nerve as the baby's head puts pressure on it.

You might think that women who have caesarian sections
won't have to worry about pain during sex. In fact, some women
choose a cesarean section to avoid the possibility of any damage in
their vulvovaginal area. However, studies show little difference

between rates of postpartum dyspareunia in women who had a cesarean section and those who delivered with no tears or episiotomy.[6] The reason? Hormones!

Recall from earlier chapters the importance of adequate levels of estrogen and testosterone in vulvar and vaginal tissue. Well, giving birth, a woman's estrogen level plunges faster than the stock market after a housing bubble bursts. Add breast-feeding, which further reduces estrogen levels, to the mix, and the dryness and pain you're experiencing even months after delivery begin to make more sense.[7] Here's how Katyia described sex after her son was born: "We tried three months after he was born, and it was extremely painful. The pain was within the vagina and during entry. Even afterwards, I felt a burning sensation for several hours. This continued for nearly a year, until I stopped nursing."

PREVENTING POSTPARTUM DYSPAREUNIA

There are ways you can reduce the risk of developing a large tear or requiring an episiotomy or the use of forceps during your delivery. The easiest way to avoid any or all of these events is by having a small baby. The size of your baby will be determined, in part, by your body mass index (BMI), a number that takes into account your weight and height. A "normal" BMI is between twenty-three and twenty-five. We recommend that you make sure you're in that range *before* you get pregnant. A BMI calculator is available at www.nhlbisupport.com/bmi.

Once the pregnancy test is positive, it's important that you stay in shape. Forget the old adage about "eating for two." You're really only eating for 1.05 (if you are having just one baby), so you don't have to increase your daily calories significantly at all. In fact, you only need about 85 more calories per day during the first trimester, 250 calories more per day during the second trimester, and 350 calories more per day during the third trimester. An apple or ba-nana has about one hundred calories. So, as you can see, the amount of food you consume doesn't have to change much.

Finally, unless your doctor or midwife recommends against it, daily moderate exercise will help maintain that healthy BMI and, at the same time, insure that your baby doesn't grow too large for an uncomplicated delivery.[8]

We also recommend that you use perineal massage to stretch your perineum in the weeks before delivery. Studies find that per-ineal massage can significantly reduce the risk of tearing or need for episiotomy during birth and pain three months after birth.[9] You should start about six weeks before your due date. You can do it yourself or invite your partner to help. Here's how:

1. Sit or lean back in a comfortable, relaxed position.
2. Smear a water-soluble lubricant like K-Y jelly or a natural oil, such as olive oil or vitamin E, on your thumb and perineum.
3. Place your thumbs about an inch inside your vagina on either side and move them in a U-shaped movement toward the rectum and to the sides, stretching the vaginal tissue and muscles and the per-ineal skin. You may feel a slight burning or stinging sensation. Over time, however, that will fade as the tissue and muscles loosen.
4. Continue for two or three minutes while breathing deeply, try-ing to relax the perineal and vaginal muscles.
5. Practice for five or ten minutes every day until delivery.

Finally, if you do wind up tearing or needing an episiotomy dur-ing childbirth, ask your doctor only to sew up the deeper layers of the perineum and to leave the skin layer unsutured. One study comparing dyspareunia rates a year after birth found women who had this type of procedure were less likely to have pain than those who had the regular procedure.[10]

PELVIC ORGAN PROLAPSE: THE HAUNTING LEGACY OF CHILDBIRTH

Another possible cause of pain during sex, one that's often related to pregnancy and childbirth, is pelvic organ prolapse (POP). The condition occurs when one or more of the organs in your pelvis—the bladder, uterus, rectum, or vagina—falls onto or into the vagina. This is often linked to tearing, during labor and delivery, of the connective tissue that surrounds your vagina and uterus and keeps the pelvic organs in place. The emerging baby tears this connective tissue and other pelvic support structures as it moves through the birth canal. Over the years, these small tears get bigger until there is an opening large enough to allow the other organs to prolapse through. The more kids you've delivered vaginally, the more likely you are to develop POP.

POP typically doesn't occur for years after your last baby. Some studies find that POP affects up to 40 percent of women aged fifty to seventy, with one study finding that of 1,000 women seeking routine gynecologic care, 76 percent had some form of POP.[11] Although childbirth is the most common cause of POP, other risk factors include abdominal pressure due to lifting, pulling, straining, and gravity, as well as chronic coughing, chronic constipation, and obesity.

POP can contribute to pain during sex in several ways:

- putting pressure on the vaginal and rectal areas
- shifting the position of the cervix
- causing tears in the vaginal tissue
- bringing irritating cervical mucus into contact with the skin of the vulva

POP can also lead to incontinence in which small amounts of urine or stool escape and irritate the vaginal area, making it sensitive to any kind of touch. In addition, the pressure and incontinence that often accompany POP can exacerbate skin disorders like lichen sclerosus and lichen planus (see Chapter 10).

(continues)

PELVIC ORGAN PROLAPSE: THE HAUNTING LEGACY OF CHILDBIRTH

(continued)

Diagnosing Pelvic Organ Prolapse

Diagnosing POP begins with a standard physical exam to look for any signs of bulging in the vaginal area. Because such bulges are less apparent when you're lying down, the exam may be performed while you're standing or squatting. The doctor will probably insert a speculum to examine the area more closely and may perform a different type of cotton swab test than you've been reading about throughout this book. Instead of lightly touching the outer part of the vagina, he or she will insert the swab into the urethra to determine how much the pelvic organs move when you strain. The doctor may also perform a rectal exam.

Treating Pelvic Organ Prolapse

Treatment for POP depends on how serious it is. For less severe cases, physical therapy to strengthen your pelvic floor, dietary and lifestyle changes to reduce constipation and its attendant straining, and pessaries, small devices you put in your vagina to support your organs, are all good options. For serious POP, surgery is the best option. The surgeon puts the organs back in place, keeping them there with an artificial mesh sling or sutures and, if necessary, repairing the prolapsed vagina. The surgery can be performed through an incision in the abdomen, laparoscopically through tiny incisions in the abdominal area, or vaginally. Most surgeries to repair POP are done vaginally, although the evidence is mixed as to which approach—abdominal or vaginal—provides the best outcome.[12] While hysterectomies are also performed in women with POP, talk to your doctor about other options first.

TREATING POSTPARTUM DYSPAREUNIA

> I enjoyed sex all through my pregnancy. But I tore quite badly
> during the delivery and had lot of stitches. I waited to have sex
> until after my six-week check up, and yes, it was very painful. I
> found that massaging the scar tissue helped a lot. And a lot of
> patience from my husband. We made sure to spend a lot of time
> with foreplay several times a week, even if we didn't have sex.
> So far, we've had sex five times, and it still hurts a lot, but after a
> few minutes, a lot of deep breaths and a lot of caressing and
> loving words from my man, the pain gets better. My advice is to
> wait until you're ready, no matter how long that takes. And re-
> member that it will start to feel better over time.
>
> —STEPHANIE, THIRTY-ONE

Stephanie is right. Numerous studies show that postpartum sexual
pain is usually temporary. In the meantime, you can do the following to ease the pain today:

- Tell your health-care professional. The six-week checkup is to
  check you out, physically and emotionally, not just to get a picture of your doctor or midwife with the baby. Even though most
  women experience pain during sex after giving birth, only 15
  percent mention it to their health-care provider.[13] That's a mis-
  take. As you learned in Chapter 3, you have to speak up when
  it comes to your sexual health. If you don't tell us there's a problem, we can't help you!
- Apply topical estrogen. You might be wondering why you can't just
  take supplemental estrogen therapy to replace the low levels contributing to your dyspareunia. The answer is that normal estrogen

blood levels reduce the quantity and quality of breast milk. However, as your baby gets older and you begin to supplement breast
milk with either formula or baby food, it is certainly possible to use
topical estrogen. If you do use this, remember to treat both the
vestibule (the opening to the vagina) and the vagina itself. We recommend using either an estrogen tablet (Vagifem) or half a gram
of estrogen cream (Estrace) in the vagina two or three times a week
and rubbing a pea-sized amount of estrogen cream on the vestibule
daily until the tenderness improves.

- Use personal lubricants. Low estrogen means low lubrication.
  That, in turn, means vaginal dryness, which translates to pain
  or, at the very least, discomfort during sex. So, we recommend
  slathering on the lubricant before intercourse. While numerous
  brands are available, we suggest saving the strawberry-flavored
  warming gel for after baby's first birthday and using instead a
  hypoallergenic brand such as Slippery Stuff or ID Moments until the hormonal changes from your pregnancy improve.

- Numb the pain. Topical anesthetics like lidocaine can numb
  frazzled nerve endings still smarting from an episiotomy or tearing. Try soaking a cotton ball in lidocaine ointment, applying it
  to the vestibule, and keeping it there overnight. One study in
  women with vulvodynia found that doing this for seven weeks
  significantly reduced the pain, enabling most women to have
  intercourse.[14] A weekly injection of a lidocaine-based solution
  in the vaginal area for three weeks can also help.

- Interfere with pain signals. If your doctor can't find any specific
  reason for your pain, such as low estrogen levels, thin vaginal tissue, or an improperly healed episiotomy or laceration, your pain
  should be treated like generalized vulvodynia (see Chapter 5).

- Try physical therapy. As with any form of sexual pain, physical
  therapy can work wonders. Specific approaches include manual
  therapy and massage, pelvic floor biofeedback, and deep ultra-

sound massage. The latter uses deep heat to promote the healing of muscles, joints, and tissues and is often used in women with pain from perineal tears.

BOTTOM LINE

If it hurts when you have sex—even if the baby has started crawling and eating solid food—don't worry! This is quite common and will improve. But if it's bothering you or your partner, talk to your doctor. As you can see from the options in this chapter, you can do several things now to relieve the pain until your body returns to its normal hormonal and physical state—a process that actually takes about a year, not the six weeks many women are led to believe.

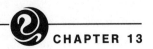

CHAPTER 13

Physical Therapy
THE UNIVERSAL TREATMENT

> The more I talked to Dr. Andrew Goldstein and the physical ther-
> apist, the more I started to realize how I was doing things sub-
> consciously but never realized it. For instance, in really stressful
> situations at work, I'd find myself all clenched up. But after a lot
> of physical therapy, particularly working on the pelvic floor mus-
> cles, I started to feel better. I learned to connect my mind and my
> physical body.
>
> —SARAH, THIRTY-TWO

W hy do we recommend physical therapy for nearly every
condition that contributes to sexual pain? Because it
works! It works because of anatomy and, as Sarah says above, because of the mind-body connection.

As Figure 13.1 shows, the pelvic floor muscles act as a kind of
hammock in the pelvis, cradling the bladder, uterus, urethra, perineum, and rectum. These muscles are quite complex. They must
contract so that you can function in the world without urinating
all the time, but relax when it's time to urinate, have a bowel
movement, or have sex. For instance, when you empty your bladder, the smooth muscle at the neck of the bladder as well as your

pelvic floor muscles should relax. But in women with interstitial cystitis or other bladder problems, the pelvic muscles actually tighten as the women strain to push out more urine. Finally, of course, the pelvic floor is involved in sexual pleasure. It enables you to tighten and relax your vagina and even plays a role in the intensity of your orgasm, with studies finding that the stronger the pelvic floor, the stronger the sensation of orgasm.[1]

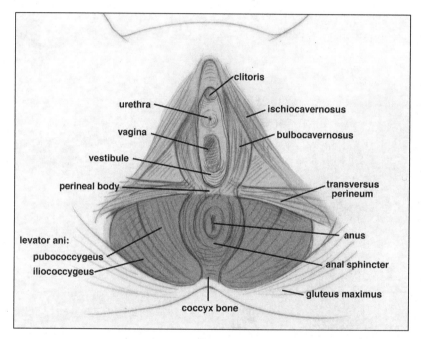

FIGURE 13.1 Female pelvic floor anatomy

There are two main types of pelvic floor dysfunction (PFD) in dyspareunia: *hypotonia*, in which the muscles are too loose (leading to problems like pelvic organ prolapse, which you learned about in Chapter 12), and *hypertonia*, in which they are overactive. The latter is the primary problem in sexual pain disorders.

That's why physical therapy is critical to the successful treatment of most causes of sexual pain. It is essential that your doctor evaluate the strength and tone (tightness) of your muscles or refer you to a physical therapist with an expertise in women's health. The studies bear this out. In one study of women with chronic vulvar pain who received physical therapy, 71 percent said their pain decreased by more than half, 62 percent said their sexual life improved, and half said their overall quality of life improved.[2] Other studies find similar or even better results.[3]

If you're too tense even to begin physical therapy, ask your doctor for a prescription for a medication like diazepam (Valium) to take before your therapy session in order to reduce your anxiety and help you relax your muscles. Your doctor can even give you a prescription for diazepam vaginal suppositories, which you can have filled at a compounding pharmacist. Taking the medication in this way limits side effects while focusing the medication's muscle-relaxing effects on the muscles that most need them.

THE PHYSICAL THERAPY EXAMINATION[4]

When you see a physical therapist, she should first conduct a full medical history and examine you. This examination involves observing how you walk, sit, lie, and move; assessing your muscle strength, tone, and endurance; and evaluating the range of motion of your joints and ligaments. The physical therapist should also check the alignment of your spine, pelvis, and neck for any abnormalities. Such structural abnormalities pull the muscles and ligaments attached to bone out of alignment, forcing other muscles to compensate. Numerous abnormal musculoskeletal conditions are associated with vulvodynia and pelvic floor dysfunction, including

- decreased mobility of the spine
- misalignment of the sacrum and the pelvis (sacroiliac dysfunction)
- a tilted pelvis, which can be caused by uneven leg lengths, muscle contractures around the hips, or a misaligned spine (pelvic obliquity)
- misalignment of the pubic bones, usually because of trauma from childbirth

Even chronic low back or hip pain can lead to overly tight pelvic muscles simply by changing the way you walk and move.

The physical therapist will also conduct an internal exam to assess the strength, mobility, and tone of your pelvic muscles. She will carefully insert a finger into your vagina without touching the vestibule. She will then press on each muscle of the pelvic floor to see if it is in spasm and identify any knots, trigger points, or tender points. She will ask you to contract (squeeze) your muscles and see how long you can hold that contraction. She will then see if you can relax your muscles. She will also palpate (gently press) the pudendal nerve and the pelvic organs to look for tenderness and mobility and to check that they are properly located.

WHAT DO I HAVE?

While you may have already been diagnosed with vulvodynia, you may get another diagnosis from your physical therapist. The names vary—pelvic floor dysfunction, levator ani syndrome, pelvic floor tension myalgia, vaginismus, anismus, coccydynia, sphincter dyssynergia, pelvic floor spasm, and a shortened pelvic floor—but all mean the same thing: too-tight, clenched, sometimes spasmed muscles. We typically use the term *pelvic floor dysfunction* and will refer to it by the acronym "PFD" throughout the rest of this chapter.

THE STORY BEHIND TIGHT MUSCLES AND SEXUAL PAIN

Pelvic floor muscles get tight for many reasons. For example, if you experience chronic vulvar pain because of lichen sclerosus, generalized vulvodynia, or chronic yeast infections, you often clench the muscles of the pelvic floor—it's a natural guarding mechanism. However, there are numerous other, less obvious causes of PFD. For instance, I (Andrew) recently treated Kristen, a twenty-four-year-old preschool teacher, with severe PFD. She developed the condition because she couldn't leave her students alone during the day, so she couldn't go to the restroom. She squeezed her pelvic floor muscles (often for eight hours a day) to "hold it in," and the muscles spasmed.

Improper exercises can also cause PFD. I have seen at least a dozen Pilates instructors who end up with PFD because they inadvertently cause spasm of their pelvic floor muscles while strengthening their cores. Finally, women who have very stressful jobs often "hold in their stress" and subconsciously squeeze their pelvic floor muscles, resulting in PFD (they also tend to tighten the muscles of their neck and shoulders, causing tension headaches and neck pain).

However, whether the spasmed muscles came first, causing the sexual pain, or the sexual pain eventually led to chronic muscle clenching and spasms doesn't really matter at this point. The reality is that this constant clenching and muscle tightening has changed the very physiology of your muscles by compressing blood vessels and limiting the flow of blood and oxygen. This, in turn, has led to a buildup of lactic acid, the same circumstances that cause muscle cramps when you exercise too intensely. In addition, those hypertonic muscles can compress nerves in the pelvic area, such as the pudendal nerve, creating pain.

THE PHYSICAL THERAPIST'S TOOLS

Physical therapists have numerous tools and treatments to relieve the tightness and spasms of the pelvic floor muscles (or to strengthen pelvic muscles as needed). One of the most basic is education. Educating you about your pelvic and structural anatomy and malfunctions in that anatomy can help you feel more in control of your situation, which can help reduce pain—or, at the very least, your perception of the pain. Other tools and methods your therapist may use are described below.

Pelvic floor surface electromyography (sEMG) biofeedback. Biofeedback is a process in which you learn to control autonomic functions like tensing or relaxing smooth muscle (often not under your direct control), changing blood flow, and even dilating blood vessels. You learn this control by seeing the muscles at work thanks to small electrodes that transmit electrical signals from the muscles to a screen. Viewing the activity helps you learn the motions and feelings required to control the activity voluntarily.

Pelvic floor sEMG is used to assess the electrical activity and tone of your pelvic muscles during the initial evaluation by a physical therapist. But the therapist also uses it to treat PFD. It doesn't hurt! You lie on the table, covered with a sheet or robe. The therapist places an internal sensor within your vagina and/or stick-on sensors on your abdomen (if you prefer to put the probe into your vagina yourself, just let the therapist know). The sensors monitor the electrical activity of the muscles, transmitting it onto the screen in the form of a graph. You can see the graph change as you tighten and relax your muscles. Over time, you learn how to elicit the muscular changes even without looking at the screen.

Each session lasts about fifty minutes but you will also be given exercises to do at home. Studies find the combination reduces the pain of vulvodynia in at least half of all women. But if you don't do the home-based exercises along with the weekly therapy, sEMG doesn't work nearly as well.[5]

Myofascial release. The fascial system is a sheath of connective tissue that covers the organs, bones, muscles, and nerves—every internal structure, actually—of your body like a single sheet of cling wrap. In a healthy system, the sheet moves with the underlying organs, muscles, and other structures. But trauma, inflammation, scarring, and even poor posture can cause the fascia to "stick" to underlying structures, reducing flexibility and stability.

In myofascial release, the physical therapist stretches and massages the muscles ("myo" means muscles) and fascia to relax and lengthen the pelvic floor. Myofascial release increases blood flow to the targeted areas. The extra oxygen and nutrients from the increased blood flow help heal the tissue and release lactic acid.

Myofascial trigger point release. In some instances, you may have trigger points, or extremely tender nodules within a tight band of muscle. These nodules occur as a result of overuse, trauma, or inflammation. Muscles with trigger points are usually contracted, weak, and hypertonic with limited range of motion. You may not even know that a trigger point is causing your pain until the physical therapist presses on it.

Physical therapists employ a variety of manual therapies to release and lengthen the muscle, using their fingers, knuckles, or even elbows to apply direct pressure on the nodule and surrounding muscle. Your doctor can also help. Physicians can inject anesthetics such as lidocaine directly into the trigger points to reduce tenderness so that the physical therapist can apply more stretching pressure without causing severe pain. In addition, an injection of botulinum toxin (Botox), which temporarily paralyzes muscle, can help, enabling the physical therapist to stretch the muscle more easily so it returns to its original length.

Connective tissue (visceral) manipulation. Here, gentle massage is used to release adhesions and spasms of the ligaments and organs in the abdomen and pelvis to return them to their natural position. About one-third of physical therapists use this technique for women with both PVD and GVD, with studies finding the approach improves symptoms by 71 percent and sexual function by 62 percent.[6]

Neural mobilization. This form of physical therapy uses various massage techniques to stretch muscles, ligaments, fascia, and scar tissue to release trapped nerves that may cause neuropathic pain.

Joint mobilization. With this approach, the therapist applies pressure to the pelvic joints and surrounding soft tissue to return normal movement and reduce pain. The pain may be the result of an abnormally tipped pelvis, unusual pressure on the pelvic joints, loss of range of motion in the hip joint, or one legs being longer than the other.

Spinal core stabilization. If you've ever taken a Pilates class or worked with an exercise trainer to stabilize your core, then you get the idea of spinal core stabilization. The goal is to strengthen the spinal, gluteal, and abdominal muscles to restore balance and strength at the pelvic base, which supports the rest of the trunk. A weak core can lead to bad posture, in turn putting stress on joints, muscles, and nerves and leading to inflammation and pain. Expect numerous exercises—including the ubiquitous abdominal crunches—to improve your core strength. It is important, however, that you do Pilates with a very experienced instructor because, as mentioned above, if done improperly, the exercises can cause spasm of the pelvic floor muscles.

Pelvic floor retraining. This approach focuses on the pelvic floor muscles themselves. Therapists use a variety of techniques and exercises, including Kegels (in which you clench and release the muscles that control the flow of urine) to strengthen pelvic floor muscles; dilators and vibrators to relax and stretch perineal and coital muscles; and sEMG biofeedback to loosen overly tight muscles and improve overall muscular control.

Electrical stimulation. This technique uses electrical current to stimulate muscles and improve their responsiveness. For sexual pain, the stimulator probe may be inserted into the vagina, or the stimulators may be placed on the pelvis. It doesn't hurt; you just feel a slight, fairly pleasant buzzing sensation.

Therapeutic ultrasound. In this procedure, an ultrasound wand uses sound waves to provide deep heat to injured tissues, such as those damaged during childbirth. The heat stimulates blood flow, improving healing.

FINDING A PELVIC FLOOR PHYSICAL THERAPIST

Finding a physical therapist trained in the techniques discussed above may not be as easy as finding a therapist to work on an injured knee or shoulder. One resource is the American Physical Therapy Association, which has a website to help find a pelvic floor physical therapist (www.womenshealthapta.org). If this website does not list a physical therapist in your area, call a local urologist or urogynecologist; they frequently refer patients to women's health physical therapists. The National Vulvodynia Association (www.nva.org) also has a list of pelvic floor physical therapists available to members.

BOTTOM LINE

As we said at the beginning of this chapter, physical therapy is an important component of any treatment plan for dyspareunia, no matter what the cause. It's not a quick-fix solution, however; it will take time to work, and you have to do your homework! But together with quality medical care and the behavioral therapy you'll read about in the next chapter, physical therapy will improve your pain and your sex life.

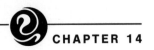

CHAPTER 14

Cognitive Behavioral Therapy

WORKING IT OUT IN YOUR HEAD

L ike physical therapy, cognitive behavioral therapy (CBT) should be an important part of any treatment plan for your pain—to help you not only with the pain itself but also with the ramifications of the pain on your relationships and life. First, a few words about CBT: It is not the type of therapy in which you lie on a couch several times a week and dissect your dreams and your relationship with your mother. Instead, CBT is based on the idea that how you think about things directly affects how you feel about them and that your inner thoughts, not external situations like people or even your pain, are related to how you feel and behave. It is a limited-time therapy, typically lasting for ten to twelve sessions, with each session highly structured and focused on a particular area.

A major goal of CBT is to change how you think about your pain in order to change how the pain feels. For instance, you may think that you've done something to cause the pain you feel or that you will never feel better. A therapist trained in CBT can help you learn to change that inner dialogue. He will help you see that your pain is related to an underlying physical condition, not to anything you've done. He will help you objectively rate your pain so you can see that it isn't constant but does ebb. If you're certain that you'll never again be sexually intimate with your partner because of the pain, he can help you identify other ways to be intimate and understand that sexual intimacy should be considered separately and apart from the pain.

Studies find that CBT can be as effective as medication for a variety of mental health conditions, including mood, anxiety, personality, and substance abuse disorders. Studies also find it is quite effective for sexual pain. In one study conducted at McGill University in Canada, seventy-eight women with vestibulodynia were randomly assigned to treatment either with CBT or biofeedback for twelve weeks or with vulvar vestibulectomy (surgery to remove nerve endings in the vulvar vestibule). Although the women undergoing surgery had significantly greater improvements in pain than women in the other two groups, women who had CBT reported significant reductions in pain and improved sexual function and psychological status.[1] After two and a half years, the women in the CBT and surgery groups had equivalent decreases in their pain, indicating that the effects of CBT are as good as those of surgery but may take more time to emerge.[2]

We have also had great success using CBT as part of the comprehensive management approach including either individual or group counseling that we advocate for our patients with dyspareunia. No matter which type of counseling our patients choose, the goals are the same. They include helping you to

- view dyspareunia as a multidimensional pain problem influenced by cognitive, emotional, behavioral, and relationship factors.

- change the factors that influence your pain so you can cope better and so the pain is not as intense. For instance, we work on our patients' tendency to catastrophize, in which women tend to view their pain as all encompassing.
- improve the quality of your sexual functioning either alone or with your partner.
- shift the focus of sexuality away from intercourse toward the pleasure available in other sexual activities.
- reduce the tendency to avoid physical intimacy and anything remotely sexual.
- adhere to other parts of your management plan, such as taking medications, doing physical therapy, and even undergoing a gynecologic exam without severe anxiety.

THE REALITY OF COGNITIVE BEHAVIORAL THERAPY[3]

Going through the therapy taught me to view even little successes as successes. Before, I was a very all-or-nothing person. But I learned to stop catastrophizing. That's one of the things the therapist drilled into us: that the negative thoughts are a downward spiral you get your mind into, and you have to stay out of that. To learn to be aware of my thoughts and feelings and think positively and constructively, and to not feel discouraged or that it was my fault, or that I was completely alone, was really important.

—KIMBERLY, THIRTY-ONE

So what is CBT like? The first step is finding a therapist trained in CBT (see "Finding a Cognitive Behavioral Therapist"). Keep in mind, however, that not all cognitive behavioral therapists deal with pain, and even fewer deal with both pain and sexuality. It's possible that you will need to find a health-care professional to help you with your pain and then seek help from a sex therapist for issues related to your sexuality.

During the first meeting, you and your therapist should discuss the therapy itself, its goals, and your personal goals. A major part of CBT is education—about your condition, the therapy, and treatments. The therapist will teach you about your condition, whether it is interstitial cystitis, vestibulodynia, or irritable bowel syndrome, including symptoms, prevalence, causes, and potential treatment. Some therapists keep a model of the pelvis in their office so that they can help you visualize what's going on with your body. Even giving you this book to read could be part of your

FACT OR FICTION?
MYTHS ABOUT PAIN

The following are two prevalent myths. How many do you believe? Take this list with you to discuss with your therapist.

1. If doctors can't cure your pain or find out exactly what is causing it, your pain must be imaginary. Not true. While pain is, of course, in your head (because that's where the brain resides, and pain is translated in the brain), it is not imaginary; it is very real. Besides, as you learned in Chapter 2, the average doctor is not terribly good at diagnosing or treating sexual pain.
2. If you can reduce your pain through psychological self-control, then the pain was "all in your head" to begin with. Not true: Pain is a private, individual experience, and many things besides the intensity of the stimulation contribute to the perception of pain (for more on this, refer back to Chapter 2).[4]

therapist's educational approach, as could listing and then debunking common myths about pain.

Through this process, the therapist will help validate your pain—in other words, she will reassure you that no matter what you've been told by other medical professionals or by your friends, family, and partner, your pain is real, not "all in your head." Part of this process involves thinking about how different situations and experiences change your perception of the pain, a process that will eventually help you feel that you have more control or power over it so that you're no longer a helpless bystander. In other words, you will control the pain; the pain won't control you.

EXERCISE 4: WHERE DOES IT HURT?

Among the exercises the therapist may do with you is one called localization. This is important because often women feel the pain has taken over their entire body when, in actuality, it is limited to one area. Here's how you can "localize" your pain:

- Locate the most painful area yourself with your fingers or a cotton swab.
- Draw a picture of your genitals, and put a star in the very spot where the pain lives.
- Bring your picture to your next therapy appointment to discuss with your therapist.

You will also learn to be realistic about your current management plan. For instance, you will realize that even if the pain isn't completely gone, an improvement of even 50 percent could make a tremendous difference in the quality of your life. Most importantly, however, you will learn that no "magic pill" or procedure exists to make the pain quickly disappear.

Your therapist should also educate you about pain itself and its effects on every aspect of a person's life, from sleep to mood. To help you view your pain more objectively, the therapist may ask you to keep a pain diary in which you rate your pain on a scale of zero to ten (zero being no pain and ten being the worst pain you've ever experienced) and to record what you were doing or thinking at the time of the pain. This is important because it helps you better understand your pain and what influences it. Simply seeing it recorded on paper, with numerical ratings, will help you view your pain more objectively. (You will find a pain diary in the "Resources" section of the appendix.) You will also learn how your own thoughts and actions may be making the pain worse. Once those thoughts are identified, the therapist will work with you to change them so they no longer have such influence over your pain and your perception it.

Other aspects of your therapy may include the following:

- Relaxation techniques. These include deep breathing exercises, focused visualization (in which you picture in your mind a place that makes you feel happy and relaxed and focus on it rather than the pain), and progressive muscle relaxation (in which you tense and then relax each muscle in your body, beginning at your toes and working your way up to your head). These exercises trigger what's called the relaxation response, slowing your heart rate, lowering your blood pressure, and reducing the release of stress hormones. They are important both to prevent anxiety when the pain occurs and to help you relax as you and your partner try to reintroduce sexuality and physical intimacy back into your lives.

- Self-coping statements. The goal of these statements is to help you develop an active rather than a passive attitude toward your pain problem. Self-coping statements might take the following forms:

  ▸ When you're worrying about the pain, remind yourself that worrying won't help. Ask yourself what you can do instead that might help (e.g., putting a frozen bag of vegetables over your vulvar area, applying topical lidocaine, taking a warm bath, and so forth).

  ▸ When you're feeling anxious that the pain might get worse, reassure yourself that this is a natural feeling but then practice your deep breathing and other relaxation exercises to dissipate the anxiety instead of letting it gain control of you.

  ▸ When you're feeling tense, remind yourself that the feeling signals that it's time to take some deep, cleansing breaths and concentrate on relaxing thoughts.

  ▸ When you start to feel overwhelmed with the pain, the doctor visits, the medical treatments, or the problems with your partner, just stop for a moment. Say to yourself, "I won't get overwhelmed. I'll just take one step (one hour, one day) at a time."

  ▸ When you feel a lot of pain, remind yourself that you have control over your body and tell yourself that you are not going to relinquish that control to the pain. Instead, concentrate on arousing fantasies and relax by breathing deeply.

  ▸ When the negative thoughts threaten to overwhelm, say to yourself, "Stop! I'm going to concentrate on the strategies my therapist and I have developed to help me cope with the pain."

HOW DO YOU BREATHE?

Perhaps it seems kind of ridiculous to think that you may need to learn how to breathe. But the reality is that most of us breathe incorrectly. We breathe shallowly, using only our chest, instead of deeply, involving our diaphragm and abdomen.

How do you breathe? To find out, lie down in a quiet place. Now place your one hand on your chest and one on your abdomen. Breathe normally and watch what happens. Does your chest rise or your abdomen? Now breathe in through your nose as deeply as possible until you feel your abdomen rise under your hand. Slowly breathe out—also through your nose—until your abdomen falls. This is the kind of deep breathing that can elicit the relaxation response.

To learn how to do diaphragmatic breathing, as it's called, follow these steps:

1. Lie down in a quiet place where you won't be interrupted.
2. Place your hands just below your belly button.
3. Close your eyes and imagine a balloon inside your abdomen.
4. Each time you breathe in, imagine the balloon filling with air. Each time you breathe out, imagine the balloon collapsing.
5. Practice for five minutes several times a day.

COGNITIVE BEHAVIORAL THERAPY AND SEX

In addition to educating you about your medical condition, your therapist will also discuss with you how the pain affects desire, arousal, and orgasm, as well as your current and past relationships. This is an important part of CBT: understanding if and why you're avoiding sexual activities, what role you play in the avoidance, and what role your partner plays. The two of you might explore the following questions:

- How do you avoid sex?
- Do you have unrealistic beliefs about or less adaptive attitudes toward sex?
- Why do you avoid sex (besides pain, of course)?
- Are there activities you can engage in that aren't painful?
- Is masturbation an option?

Together, you and your therapist will work through potential solutions so that you and your partner can maintain the physical intimacy we discussed in Chapter 4, even if you're not having intercourse.

Your therapist may also recommend desensitization exercises. This could involve watching a video of women masturbating to help you learn to view your genital area again as something that

FINDING A COGNITIVE BEHAVIORAL THERAPIST

The following organizations can help you locate a therapist trained and/or accredited or certified in CBT:

National Association of Cognitive Behavioral Therapists (NACBT)
www.nacbt.org

Association of Behavioral and Cognitive Therapies (ABCT)
www.abct.org

Academy of Cognitive Therapy (ACT)
www.academyofct.org

The National Vulvodynia Association (NVA)
www.nva.org

can give pleasure, not just pain. Plus, masturbation is a good sexual activity to bring back into your life because you have total control over it, and it will help awaken your dormant libido.

Another desensitization exercise involves using a vaginal dilator to break the association between having something inside your vagina and pain. So, you may be asked to practice your relaxation or breathing exercises once a day while you gently and slowly insert something into your vagina. It could initially be as small as your little finger; later, it might be a larger finger, then a carrot or zucchini (covered with a condom).

BOTTOM LINE

As you can see, CBT is a complex, yet highly effective, approach that will help you gain control over the pain. And control, in and of itself, will reduce your pain—we promise! Like physical therapy, however, CBT takes time and practice to be effective. Expect homework assignments, and make sure you do them. Remember, you're retraining your brain to think differently about your pain. That takes just as much practice as retraining your body to be able to run in a marathon.

PART III

When the Pain Is Gone

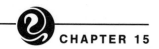

CHAPTER 15

Rebuilding Your Life

So, the pain is gone (or, at least, it's much, much better). You're starting to feel like you've got your life back—to recognize the old you, the person with energy and the ability to focus on something other than pain. You're even beginning to—gasp!—feel the first tender shoots of desire. So, you think, you'll head to the bedroom with your husband (or boyfriend or partner), and everything will be just like it used to be, only better.

Not so fast.

You have to understand that you don't simply "get over" the kind of psychological and physical trauma you've experienced (often for years) as if it were nothing more than a trifling hangnail. That's because it isn't simply that you were experiencing pain; you were the pain. You weren't sexual or maternal or wifely or motherly or anything else because there was no room in your life for you to be anything other than someone who hurt.

Yes, we're sure you're quite happy to walk away from that persona and don another. But we can tell you, based on our cumulative thirty plus years of experience, it's not that simple. Although the only thing you've wanted, the goal of your work over the past months, has been to vanquish the pain, I bet you didn't realize that in the process you'd also be vanquishing a part—albeit a small one—of yourself.

This is perfectly normal. For so long the pain circumscribed your life, trapping you in a tight little box from which you fought to escape. It defined your life, determining the type of relationship you could have with your partner, the physical and sexual activities you could perform, and your ability to feel joy and pleasure. Before you can really return to the "old" you, you have to let go of the enormous presence of the pain in your life and learn—yes, learn, just as a preschooler learns her alphabet—to realize that other issues exist. This is a hard shift to make—but then again, most things in life worth having are challenging. Why should remaking yourself be any exception?

MAKING THE SHIFT

So, how do you make the shift? Unfortunately, we can't provide a magic formula or recipe. Each woman is different, depending on her individual situation.

Take Amy, twenty-eight, whose dyspareunia began about seven years ago. At the time, she was in a serious relationship with a man she loved. Her problem began with dryness and burning pain, accompanied by chronic yeast infections. Eventually, the pain grew so bad that she lost interest in sex altogether. She was eventually diagnosed with lichen planus. Even with treatment, the pain continued.

Her boyfriend was no help. "He wasn't horrible," she says, "but he wasn't supportive." The relationship ended so badly that it left her leery of future relationships. Eventually she found her way to me (Caroline) and enrolled in our study of pelvic floor physiotherapy combined with biofeedback and group cognitive behavioral therapy sessions. The combination clicked, and Amy began to recover.

During this time, she met a new man. As her pain resolved, Amy worked with her therapist to explain to this new man what she'd been through and how her sexual pain had affected her emotionally as well as physically. The two waited six months to have intercourse, and while "it wasn't wonderful, it was better" than sex had been before, Amy said.

The two had a long-distance relationship, so sex occurred sporadically. But it kept getting better, as did the relationship. One reason? Amy continued therapy even after her pain dissipated. Her therapist helped her deal with her fears about sex and a new relationship, with the stresses of a long-distance romance, and when her boyfriend proposed, with her anxiety about marriage. We are happy to report that Amy is now happily married and living overseas with her husband, and both of them are doing quite well.

The message we want you to take away from this story is that Amy didn't just focus on getting rid of the pain; she realized that she was going to need some help repairing the damage that the pain had done to her confidence and psyche. So, if you've been involved in therapy as part of your pain management program (as we recommend strongly throughout this book, particularly in Chapter 14 on cognitive behavioral therapy), we urge you to continue. You will need the support of a good therapist as you reenter the world of the pain-free.

HOW YOU CAN MAKE POSITIVE CHANGE: AN EXERCISE

Now we want you to do a little exercise. We promise it won't hurt! Carve out an hour or two when you know you won't be interrupted or distracted. Turn off your cell phone, and make yourself comfortable. Now think. Think about where you are in your life and where you'd like to be. What positive changes do you want to make in your life and relationship? Write them down.

Now, look at each change and ask yourself, "How will I get there?" For instance, if you'd like to rediscover your libido, how do you plan to do it? It's not as if it's buried in the detritus at the bottom of your closet, you know. You have to actively entice it back. The next chapter, "When Sex Is Good," provides some ideas.

We've also seen our patients make other positive changes:

- Improving their relationships. There's no getting around the damage dyspareunia wreaks on even the healthiest of relationships (return to Chapter 4 if you don't believe us). We strongly recommend some couples therapy or, at the very least, that the two of you carve out regular time to focus on each other and your relationship, including taking a trip away, if possible. For some couples, this period becomes like a second honeymoon, one of experimentation and risk taking as they relearn each other's bodies (see next page for more on relationships).

- Increasing their physical activity levels. As you know, vulvar pain can make exercising, even walking, out of the question. Now that you're feeling better, it's time to return to the gym, lace up your running shoes, or even dust off your bike and hit the open road—things you may have thought you'd never do again.

- Having a baby. For women with vulvar pain, the idea of sex is bad enough—but to push out a baby? Fuggedaboutit. Well, now that sex is back in the picture, it might be time to reconsider the whole parenthood thing. If your cycle is regular, and everything is working with you and your partner, there is no reason why you can't get pregnant and have a baby (or two, or more!). If you are on any medications or undergoing any form of treatment, consult your doctor first to be sure you have the green light. (For more information on pregnancy, delivery, and much,

much more, please consult the "Vulvodynia, Pregnancy and Childbirth" guide available through the National Vulvodynia Association at www.nva.org.)

- Following a dream. With the pain gone, many of our patients feel as if they have a new lease on life. It reminds them of the brevity of life and provides them with the courage to take on new challenges, whether that's climbing a mountain, starting a cupcake business, or returning to law school.

COMMUNICATING NEEDS IN THE RELATIONSHIP

Let's talk a bit more about the relationship issue. As you continue healing, remember that your partner is also healing. So now, more than ever, is a time to maintain open communication—about everything. We also encourage you to experiment a bit in the bedroom. You may find that things that worked in the past no longer work to turn you on and bring you to orgasm. You may have to find a "new normal" when it comes to intimacy and sex. That's a good thing; it keeps the relationship fresh!

As you work through various issues with your partner, keep in mind what you learned about the relationship during your period of pain. For one, if you're still together, you learned that the two of you can survive a serious health issue. This is really an amazing thing; so often we see relationships crumble under the weight of dyspareunia or even far less serious medical issues. The fact that the two of you survived means that you will have the strength to handle other challenges life throws at you, from financial setbacks to children.

Conversely, if you feel that the experience you've just been through weakened your relationship, it might be time to reexamine it, to look at it with fresh eyes. Is this the partner you want for the long term? Will he be able to give you what you need if and when other challenges arise (and trust us, they will arise!). If not, and if you don't feel that the two of you can repair the damage, it might be time to leave.

Now do you understand why we think it's so important that you keep seeing your therapist?

WHEN THE PAIN ISN'T GONE

Sometimes, you may find that while the pain is much better, it's still there, albeit to a lesser degree. The reality is that you may have to learn to live with some level of pain. If this occurs, don't become discouraged. The fact that the pain is much reduced should greatly improve your overall quality of life. We also want you to continue working with your medical team—the therapists, physicians, and others who got you to this point. Remember from the previous section: Sometimes it can take years of work before the pain resolves.

BOTTOM LINE

The bottom line from this chapter, the nugget we want you to take away, is that you have the opportunity to take the first step into the rest of your life. Take advantage of it to create new experiences for yourself and your partner through what you have learned about yourself and your relationship.

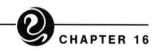

CHAPTER 16

When Sex Is Good

The women who come to see us are in more than just physical pain; they are also in psychological pain because they can no longer enjoy a normal sexual relationship. As with many things, you just don't realize how important sex is to a relationship, your sense of self, and your overall happiness and contentment until it's gone. As April, thirty-two, told us:

> I enjoy being with my husband. Sex is very important for him as it is one of his primary ways to express his love. When I cannot provide a way for him to do that, it is very frustrating for me. Sometimes I feel inadequate as a woman that I cannot provide this for him. He is understanding and helpful but that does not change the fact that a major part of our marriage is compromised. Sure, we can cuddle and do other things to please one another without intercourse, but it is not the same. I believe and look forward to the day that this issue is not a part of our relationship and that we can enjoy a normal sex life without my physical pain.

April at least remembers what having a normal sex life felt like. But many of the women we see have experienced pain since the very first time they tried to have intercourse. So they have no idea what a "normal" sex life is like. Or they've been coping with pain and torment for so long that they no longer remember pleasurable sex.

That's why we've included this chapter. We want to remind you of (or educate you about) fun, passionate, thrilling sex *that feels good*. We also want to dispel some myths about sex that, whether you realize it or not, may have contributed (or be contributing) in some small way to where you've been sexually and where you are now, with the pain gone or, at the very least, much improved.

DEFINING "NORMAL"

> What people don't realize is that when you have genital pain, it's not the same thing as pain in your arm or leg. You can't detach yourself from it in the same way as a broken arm because a broken arm isn't so fundamental to who you are. Plus, not being able to have sex is defeminizing. I felt that if this part of me didn't work like it should, then I was less of a woman.
> —MARCY, THIRTY-THREE

Read any women's magazine, and it seems that not only are women everywhere having sex several times a day, but they're having incredible sex, complete with multiple orgasms. We've got news for you: This is not reality. Instead, it is some kind of Hollywood version of sex. Reality is scheduling sex because between the kids, the job, and the chores, there is not enough time for such intimacy. Reality is waking up one day and realizing that you haven't had sex in over a month. Reality is lying there after sex wondering if he'll hear if you masturbate yourself to orgasm. Reality is sex that's satisfying but that lasted about a minute. Reality is wondering why he wants it all the time and you don't.

However, reality may also be feeling a tingling throughout your entire body every time your partner touches you, aching to feel him inside and on top of you, fantasizing about lovemaking in all its potential. In other words, there is no "normal." Normal is what feels right for you.

SEXUAL MYTHS AND REALITIES

Now, let's look at some common myths we've found that our patients (those with and without pain) often hold about sex in the twenty-first century.

Myth. Everyone is having more sex than me.

Reality. Women in their twenties through forties have sex, on average, between one and eleven times a month.[1]

Myth. Intercourse is a required part of lovemaking.

Reality. For some reason, society has determined that penetration is the apex of sex. This is one reason the women we see feel so much shame about their inability to have "normal" sex. They feel that if they're not having penetrative intercourse, then something really big is missing, and intimacy with their partner is over. These women have decided that the sensation of having their partner inside them (or, in the case of men, being inside their partner) is so fulfilling and satisfying that nothing else can compare. But the reality is that penetrative intercourse is not the be all and end all of good sex or intimacy.

Yes, intercourse can be fabulous, but it does not have to be a syn-onym for sex. In fact, when researchers at the Kinsey Institute in Bloomington, Indiana, asked six hundred undergraduate students to define sex, 19 percent did not consider penile-vaginal intercourse as the only type of sex. Students also listed "deep kissing," "breast con-tact," "manual stimulation of the genitals," and "oral-genital" con-tact as sex.[2] A whole world of sexuality and sensuality out there can count as sexual above and beyond physical intercourse. You learned about this in Chapter 4; if you're not ready for intercourse, revisit that chapter to remind yourself about other ways to be intimate.

Myth. Married people always have sex.

Reality. One of the first large-scale studies to evaluate the fre-quency of sex among married couples analyzed a sample of 6,029 married people from the National Survey of Families and House-holds. The researchers wanted to learn about sexual frequency. They found that 16 percent of the couples had not had sex in the month before the interview. It is important to keep in mind that there is a huge variation in terms of frequency of sex![3]

Myth. If I don't reach orgasm, the sex failed.

Reality. In a national survey of women, just one-third thought that orgasm was important for sexual satisfaction.[4] Other studies find that just one-third of women say they regularly have orgasms dur-ing vaginal sex (and, in fact, vaginal sex is the least effective way to reach orgasm). And while there are certain reasons for an inabil-ity to orgasm—medications, hormonal changes—every woman is capable of doing so. So yes, while important, orgasm should not be-come the epitome of sex. Nor should your sexual pleasure be judged solely on whether you attained climax.

Sex, with or without orgasm, can feel fabulous, but if you are expecting mind-blowing orgasms each and every time you have sex, you'll probably be disappointed. The downside of such high expectations is that if the single goal of orgasm is not reached, it negatively colors the rest of the activity; you may ignore or down-play the other great parts of sex. Plus, the more you focus on having an orgasm, the less likely you are to have one! That's because

ORGASM DEFINED

Here's an interesting question for you. If you've never had an orgasm, how do you know when you are having one? This is kind of like the pornography question that the Supreme Court addressed years ago: You'll know it when you see (feel) it. Actually, certain physical road signs nearly always occur with orgasm:

- tingling that may begin in your vaginal/pelvic area but soon spreads throughout your body, increasing in intensity
- a sense of peaking, as if you are riding a rollercoaster and have reached the top of the first ascent, where you hang, for just a moment, before hurtling down
- a series of intense vaginal/pelvic/uterine contracts that may even extend into your anal region (don't be embarrassed if you pass gas)

Having said that, some women say they orgasm without any contractions. Maybe the best sign that you've had an orgasm is how you feel afterward: relieved, spent, relaxed, and calm. You have an overall sense of well-being, stimulated in part by release of the feel-good hormone oxytocin, which occurs during orgasm.

Once you've orgasmed, however, you don't have to stop. Continued stimulation, whether from your partner or yourself, can lead to rearousal and another orgasm. How many? According to those famous sexologists William Masters and Virginia Johnson, up to six an hour.

your focus on the goal of orgasm means you can't relax and sink into the sensations of sex that ultimately lead to orgasm. It's kind of a mind over body thing, and this is definitely one of those times where body takes precedence over mind.

Myth. Only clitoral stimulation can lead to orgasm.

Reality. While clitoral stimulation is the most common route to an orgasm, women can have orgasms while stimulating the vagina, the G-spot within the vagina, the vestibule, the mons pubis, and even the breasts and nipples. There are even reports of orgasm occurring in women after someone blew on their hair! Some women can even reach orgasm through fantasy alone. And if you've ever had a vividly sexual dream, then you know that orgasm can occur even while you are asleep. Obviously, then, your brain has as much to do with orgasm as your body.

Myth. Faking an orgasm is okay.

Reality. This is so not true! For one, if you fake an orgasm, then your partner will think whatever he did worked and that he should keep doing it. If it didn't feel good and didn't bring you to orgasm, you're stuck. And two, do you really want to build an intimate relationship on the basis of a lie?

Myth. When the passion in a relationship fades, so does the relationship.

Reality. If you tried to maintain the twice-a-day, everywhere-in-the-house sex that often marks a new romantic relationship, you'd literally love yourself into an early grave. Scientists who study the brains of couples in the throes of such passion report little activity in areas related to critical thought,[5] while others describe brain activity during such phases of passion as "mental chaos."[6] After all, if the sex is explosive, why would you need (or want) to evaluate your partner critically?

Only when the passion begins to wane, whether out of exhaustion, familiarity, or other issues, does the relationship transition from passionate love to, if you're lucky, what some experts call "companionate" love, the type that sustains a relationship over months, years, and decades. This is the type of love you need for a long-term, solid relationship. It allows you to explore previously unexplored areas of your sexuality because you can trust this other person so completely. While passionate love begins and ends with the physical, companionate love is deeply rooted in other components, including friendship, trust, similar values, and a shared life. Sex remains a part of your life, but it no longer is your life.

Myth. There's no way to recapture the heady early days of romance in the bedroom.

Reality. Sure there is! Take a trip (preferably without kids). Shedding responsibilities and experiencing a novel environment often leads to "vacation sex," as many women call it, a harkening back to those sex-soaked days of yore. Even if you can't take a physical trip, simply carving out a bit of time for the two of you without the hassles of daily life (think of an overnight in a downtown hotel) can enhance that intimacy and communication. In fact, a Canadian study found that couples who had been together for a long time actually had better sex than couples that had been together for a shorter period. The reason? They made it a priority to create time for sex with one another, to enjoy and explore their sensuality.[7]

A WOMAN IS NOT A MAN
(AND VICE VERSA)

I'd always had a very strong and high libido. When I lost that, I
felt like I lost a part of myself.

—AMY, TWENTY-EIGHT

For decades (nay, centuries), women's sexuality was explained
through a male prism; that is, a woman's sexual response was like a
man's. Like a man, she got excited thinking about sex or encoun-
tering a potential partner. As with a man, that excitement translated into a physical reaction (wetness for her, erection for him),
leading to intercourse and culminating in a sexual release.

The trailblazing sexuality researchers William Masters and Virginia Johnson used this perspective to develop their four-stage
model of sexuality in 1966:

1. Excitement: racing heart, flushed skin, erection in the male,
   engorged clitoris and labia minora in the female, as well as
   vaginal lubrication.
2. Plateau: the physical reactions of the excitement phase that
   intensify to the point of orgasm.
3. Orgasm: muscle contractions, increased blood pressure and
   heart rate, and release of sexual tension.
4. Resolution: return to a normal state. For men, it may take several
   minutes to hours to reach excitement again; women, however,
   may reach that state quite quickly, even having multiple orgasms.

Note how every phase focuses on the physical. It would be
more than ten years before the word "desire" was added to the
mix, and even then it was defined as the longing to have sex, the

to-be-expected response to excitement. For men, this is easy to understand. What man has an erection and doesn't desire sex? The reality is a bit different in women.

Around this time came the Viagrazation of sex. Suddenly, men who couldn't have sex (note: not men who didn't want sex) could swallow a little blue pill and become a bull in the bedroom. Women wanted to know where their little blue pill was. We thought we might have it in the form of therapy using testosterone, which plays a role in libido. But testosterone can deal with sexual health problems due to hormonal changes. And while several pharmaceutical companies are working on their own version of a little pink pill for women, the reality is that women's sexuality is complex, and it's doubtful any single pill will ever have the desired effect on every woman.

Here's the rub: Viagra and similar medications are designed to increase blood flow to the genitals. Just because a man or woman is physically ready for sex doesn't mean he or she wants to make love. We saw this in a study in which researchers gave women a medication to increase their genital blood flow, lubrication, and tingling sensations. If the women weren't emotionally interested in sex, however, they called this physical arousal "intrusive and unpleasant."

This study showed that there can be a disconnect between a woman's mind and her body. In order for a woman to have a satisfying sexual experience, both her mind and body have to be on the same page. That is, she must have both desire and arousal. In other words, most of the time, you need to want to have sex in order to really get into it. However, we also find that when we encourage women to consider having sex with their partner even if they're not feeling very aroused, most still report they were able to enjoy the experience. Our point is that you need to get creative and try different things with your partner, particularly now that sex is not painful.

WHY HAVE SEX?

For women, the primary motivations for having sex, beyond the desire for pregnancy, are passionate love and pleasure. Other reasons include "spiritual transcendence, duty, conformity, to improve self-esteem or status, kindness, power over another, curiosity and stress reduction."[8]

What are some of the reasons you have sex? It's worth thinking about the various reasons that led you to have sex when you were physically able to. Is it possible to meet those needs in other ways? How has your inability to have sex affected those needs? These are important questions to consider now and in the future. For as you work through your issues with painful sex and are able to begin, once again, to think of sex as a pleasurable act, it will become very important that you also assess your own reasons for wanting sex and what that means about your relationship with yourself and your partner.

Picture this. It's Wednesday night and the thought hits you: "I think I want to make love." Now, you could be thinking this due to numerous factors. Maybe your partner did the dishes and put the kids to bed, so you're feeling grateful (or at least not resentful about having to do it all yourself); maybe you feel guilty because you haven't made love in a few days; maybe you had a rough day at work and need a stress reliever; maybe your husband looks awfully good in that torn sweatshirt he wears after work. If these thoughts continue long enough and are accompanied by pleasurable sensations (a neck rub from the husband, a passionate kiss, even a good conversation), then you're ready to take things to the next level and have sex. If the sex is good, if you achieve your original goal, whatever that may be, then you've fulfilled your desire.[9]

Given all that, it becomes easier to understand why it's more complicated for a woman to become aroused and for her arousal to lead to desire. For instance, consider how the following might affect your desire:

- Lack of intimacy with your partner. The two of you have been fighting, he's been working all the time, or he's been cold and distant. Or maybe your busy lives have you both going in so many directions at the same time that you've lost the way back to each other.
- Not feeling desired or sexy. Maybe your partner only touches you when he wants sex. Or he ogles other women when you're around. Or he criticizes your appearance.
- Inability to relax enough to have sex. You're stressed for any number of reasons: The house is a mess, the kids are always underfoot, you're worried about money or getting pregnant, or work is a nightmare. Or the emotional baggage from your upbringing or previous sexual relationships keeps interfering in this relationship.
- Illness. You're tired, depressed, or sick. Or, conversely, you're taking medication such as antidepressants or birth control pills that may interfere with desire.

And, of course, there is the major issue you have experienced: pain. Whenever pain is linked with an activity, we become hardwired to begin avoiding that activity and anything that might lead up to it. This is particularly true when we talk about painful sex. The association between a potentially pleasurable event and pain can wreak havoc on your sexual response, often leading to your avoiding anything related to the possibility of sex. In women with sexual pain, we often see that the arousal and desire responses become dampened over time until, as the pain becomes more chronic, they disappear entirely. This decline may start almost imperceptibly with loss of the ability to reach orgasm. Then you notice that your ability to become wet, or lubricated, is also affected. Then we see the loss of desire. This is to be expected. If something is painful, or not pleasurable, it begins to affect all levels of response.

Even though your pain was most likely the primary reason for your reduced arousal and libido, it's important to keep other desire-killing possibilities in mind. Far too often we see women who overcome their pain only to bemoan their continued lack of desire. Quite often, it's related to other areas of conflict, areas we discussed back in Chapter 4. Ultimately, here are the most important things to keep in mind about your desire and sexual life now that the pain has improved:

1. The desire for sex may not be the most common reason you initiate or participate in sex. And that's perfectly normal.
2. Arousal or lack thereof in premenopausal women is related more to your thoughts and emotions than to any physical influences.
3. Intimacy and sex are not the same. Don't believe us? Return to Chapter 4.

Before we turn to the final chapter, we just want to stop here and say how great it is that you've made it this far in the book, whether or not your pain is actually gone. The more you know about sex, intimacy, and desire, the sooner you will rediscover all three in your life.

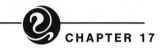

CHAPTER 17

Looking Toward the Future

Throughout this book, you've heard us say things like, "There's little evidence, but . . . ," "only a couple of studies . . . ," and "in our experience. . . . " You've also heard us talk about the many changes in our understanding of dyspareunia that have occurred just in the past few years. The reason for all this is that, medically at least, our understanding of dyspareunia is currently at about the level of our understanding of HIV and AIDS in the early 1990s. In other words, we have a long way to go.

Unfortunately, while there was a huge amount of research money available for HIV in the 1990s, there is still very little money for studies on dyspareunia. Only through science can we improve our understanding of the disorders that contribute to dyspareunia and thereby prevent the kind of doctor runaround, missed or incorrect diagnoses, and years of unnecessary pain many of our patients experience. In medicine, that means well-designed, well-conducted clinical trials, surveys, and analyses.[1]

While we applaud all the researchers who perform research on vulvar and sexual pain disorders, we cannot help but be frustrated by many of studies they produce. These clinical trials are simply not well designed. For instance, one study reported on the use of topical gabapentin (Neurontin) to treat localized and generalized vulvody-nia.[2] However, it didn't try to identify the cause of the vulvar pain before starting treatment. Wouldn't it have been better if the re-searchers excluded patients who had vulvar pain because of hor-monal causes or tight muscles and instead focused on women who had vulvar pain because of inflamed nerves? After all, you wouldn't test a treatment for angina (chest pain resulting from blocked coro-nary arteries) without first ensuring that the only people enrolled in the study actually had angina, not some other underlying cause of chest pain such as lung cancer or inflammation of the costochondral joints of the chest (the joints that link the bones in your rib cage).

Another problem with clinical trials in this area is that few are placebo controlled. The gold standard in medical research is the double-blind, randomized, placebo-controlled clinical trial. That means participants are randomly assigned to receive either the intervention (treatment) or a "fake" treatment, like a sugar pill or even "pretend" procedure, such as injections of saline instead of pain relievers to test a new analgesic. The "double-blind" part of the phrase refers to the fact that neither patients nor researchers know who receives the real treatment and who gets the placebo.

If a trial isn't placebo-controlled, then it's not very helpful be-cause we don't know if the treatment itself resulted in the response or if it was a "placebo response." The placebo response is a very real phenomenon in which the simple act of doing something, of receiv-ing attention, can actually lead to a medically valid improvement.[3] Only with a placebo-controlled arm in the trial can we learn whether the result was related to the intervention or to the placebo effect. This is particularly important in vulvodynia and vestibulody-nia because we see such a strong placebo-related effect from any in-tervention.[4] And, in fact, placebo effects are very strong in any pain treatment studies, as well as studies for other conditions with a strong cognitive component like depression and anxiety.

Don't women with vulvodynia, vestibulodynia, or other causes of dyspareunia deserve the same high level of clinical research into their conditions as those with cancer and heart disease? The problem is that for too long too much of the research in this area has been treated as an afterthought—as have the women with the conditions themselves. Okay, enough of our rant. Now let's talk about where the field is going—or, more specifically, where it needs to go in terms of research.

Better diagnosis. As you saw in Chapter 6, the diagnostic categories for provoked vestibulodynia are so unclear that I (Andrew) have taken it upon myself to develop more specific ones. However, these are the result of just one doctor's opinion. We need an established medical organization, such as the International Society for the Study of Vulvovaginal Disease (ISSVD), to refine, accept, and disseminate these categories. We also need better acceptance of the categories the ISSVD has already developed. For instance, in 1999 the ISSVD World Congress recommended replacing the term *vestibulitis* with *vestibulodynia* since, as you learned in Chapter 6, the word "vestibulitis" implies inflammation, and we know that the condition is related to far more underlying causes than inflammation alone.[5] Yet, health-care professionals who deal with sexual pain have been slow, if not downright resistant, to incorporate this word into their clinical practice.[6] This, in turn, results in different understandings of the disease, different criteria for diagnosis, and, of course, a plethora of treatments that may or may not work.

More epidemiological research. Epidemiology is the study of health in populations. It looks at likely causes or at least correlations between disease and environment. So, for instance, a study looking at the link between hormonal birth control and dyspareunia is epidemiological, as is one trying to determine how many women have dyspareunia. What's missing in many areas of sexual pain research, particularly for vulvodynia, are numbers. How many women are affected? How long does the pain last? How much does the disease cost? What is the cost-benefit ratio of various treatments? What is the overlap with other conditions, such as depression, anxiety, and other pain disorders?

Research into this overlap is particularly important since, as Chapter 9 shows, women with irritable bowel syndrome and interstitial cystitis often have vulvodynia. So do women with fibromyalgia, another chronic pain condition. Why? Early research suggests the connection may be related, among other reasons, to dysfunction in the automatic nervous system, that is, to how these women react to painful or any other kind of stimuli, or to some form of muscle dysfunction. A better understanding of the underlying pathology that links these conditions could lead to better treatments for all. The National Provider-Based Vulvodynia Outcomes Registry is the first step to significantly improving epidemiological research into vulvodynia.

More biologic research. In just the past couple of years, our understanding of the underlying pathology, or cause, of various dyspareunia-related conditions has gained ground, thanks to studies like Caroline's use of MRI to examine the brains of women with vulvodynia and to laboratory-based studies using biopsied tissue to identify molecular markers at the cellular or subcellular level related to dyspareunic conditions. We're just at the tip of the proverbial iceberg, however. We need more work on the molecular and neurological basis of these conditions if we are to develop better, more targeted treatments.

THE NATIONAL PROVIDER-BASED VULVODYNIA OUTCOMES REGISTRY

To get at some of these unanswered questions about vulvodynia, several researchers, in conjunction with the National Vulvodynia Association, have created a geographically diverse registry called the National Provider-Based Vulvodynia Outcomes Registry.[7] Information about patients with vulvodynia and vestibulodynia will be entered into the registry so that researchers can track patients through their evaluation, diagnosis, treatment, and follow-up. The goals of the registry are to

- objectively measure baseline patient characteristics, such as self-reported symptoms, pain levels, physical and sexual function, psychological distress, and quality of life
- objectively measure the level of skin and muscle sensitivity
- investigate the potential for subtypes of the disease, like the ones described in Chapters 5 and 6
- determine if adding patient characteristics to the skin and muscle measurement might better predict the outcome of commonly used treatments
- better describe the necessary components of the multidisciplinary treatment used to improve pain and quality of life
- create a multicenter network and database to generate data for larger, randomized clinical trials for various therapies

I (Andrew) am a participating provider and would encourage you to ask your doctor or clinic manager if they are participating in the registry. If they are and you feel comfortable doing it, ask for information on participating.

More randomized clinical trials on treatments. In too many instances, the treatments we use for vulvodynia and vestibulodynia are based on anecdotal evidence—that is, it worked for other patients, so it should work for you—rather than clinical evidence. We need this evidence base for our treatments not only in order to know what works and doesn't work—and thus avoid wasting time and money on ineffective treatments—but to garner insurance coverage for the treatments (few insurance companies cover treatments they consider "experimental"). We also need scientific evidence so that organizations like the ISSVD can develop and issue evidence-based guidelines for clinicians to follow in the diagnosis and treatment of these conditions.

Greater understanding of dyspareunia and relationships. We know intuitively that painful sex affects relationships and that a bad relationship can make dyspareunia worse. But we don't know as well as we should at this point how and why. More importantly, we don't know how to "inoculate" a relationship against potential damage from sexual pain and, after the pain improves, how to rehabilitate that relationship. We also need to know more about the impact of the dyspareunia on the partner, male or female.

Now let's talk a bit about some of the research that's actually occurring.[8]

Diagnosis and pathology. Researchers are looking at the ability of quantitative sensory testing, which objectively measures the effect of various sensations (hot, cold, touch, vibration), to assess neurologic problems that could be responsible for the pain. Another option is carbon dioxide laser–invoked potentials. Briefly, this device stimulates your skin with short pulses of carbon dioxide to assess the function of your pain perception system.[9] Finally, given studies that find higher levels of certain inflammatory chemicals in the blood of women with some sexual pain conditions, there may one day be a simple blood test that can assess whether you have vulvodynia or a similar condition.[10]

Treatment. To develop treatments specifically for vulvodynia and related conditions, researchers are investigating the pain-relieving properties of venom produced by carnivorous sea snails,[11] compounds derived from marijuana,[12] and molecular-based strategies to reduce the ability of cells to produce pain-producing proteins.[13] They are also looking into using functional MRI—in which you can see the effect of a stimulus on parts of your brain—as a kind of supercharged biofeedback to teach patients to control their brain's reaction to pain.[14]

YOUR ROLE

You have a role to play in future research too. Here's what you can do:

- Be vocal. Don't be ashamed of your problem. Discuss it with friends, in chat rooms, or on your blog. We all must do everything that we can to eradicate the stigma of sexual pain.
- Participate. If your physician, physical therapist, or mental health therapist asks if you'd like to participate in a clinical trial, please go the extra mile and say yes. While there are valid reasons to refuse (you could get the placebo medication for a few months, have to make a few extra visits to their office, or need an extra skin biopsy or other procedure), if you don't participate, we may never get the answers we need.

    I (Andrew) once had a grant to study the benefit of venlafaxine (Effexor) for vulvodynia. I had to return the grant money because so few women agreed to join the study. To this day, we don't know if this medication would have helped.
- Offer support. There are excellent organizations such as the National Vulvodynia Association (NVA) and the Interstitial Cystitis Association (and others listed in the "Resources" section of

the appendix) that do a great deal with very little money. When you support these organizations with donations, you help yourself and millions of women who suffer like you. That's why we will donate 25 percent of all proceeds from the sale of this book to the NVA.

BOTTOM LINE

We hope this chapter has given you, well, hope—that you can see that we are only at the beginning of what promises to be a long but fruitful journey to better understand the underlying pathology of dyspareunia-related conditions. Such an understanding will enable us to develop better ways to diagnose and treat those conditions. All it takes is time and money! We also hope that this book itself has given you hope—that you've learned from it, gained confidence in your ability to take charge of your health, and comfort in the knowledge that you don't have to suffer alone, if you can find the right health-care professional, for much longer.

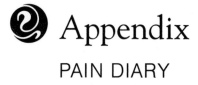 # Appendix

PAIN DIARY

Fill out this form after engaging in an activity that caused pain (e.g., intercourse, finger insertion, and so forth).

Date and time:

Time of menstrual cycle:

What activity triggered the pain?

How much pain did you feel? (Rate it on a scale of 1 to 10, with 1, 2, 3 being mild pain; 4, 5, 6 being moderate pain; 7, 8, 9 being severe pain; and 10 being the worst pain experienced.)

How long did the pain last?

What were your thoughts and feelings just prior to the pain?
During the pain? After the pain?

What was your general mood like?

If pain was triggered by sexual activity:
　　How sexually aroused were you before the pain started?

　　How lubricated were you?

What did you do to try to reduce the pain? How much did it help?

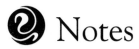 Notes

NOTES TO CHAPTER ONE

1. A. Goldstein, C. F. Pukall, and I. Goldstein, *Female Sexual Pain Disorders: Evaluation and Management* (New York: Wiley-Blackwell, 2009).

2. L. D. Arnold et al., "Vulvodynia: Characteristics and Associations with Comorbidities and Quality of Life," *Obstet Gynecol* 107, no. 3 (2006): 617–624.

3. R. Tannahill, *Sex in History* (New York: Stein and Day, 1982).

NOTES TO CHAPTER TWO

1. R. W. Hurley and M. C. Adams, "Sex, Gender, and Pain: An Overview of a Complex Field," *Anesth Analg* 107, no. 1 (2008): 309–317.

2. F. M. Levine and L. L. De Simone, "The Effects of Experimenter Gender on Pain Report in Male and Female Subjects," *Pain* 44, no. 1 (1991): 69–72.

3. K. Gijsbers and F. Nicholson, "Experimental Pain Thresholds Influenced by Sex of Experimenter," *Percept Mot Skills* 101, no. 3 (2005): 803–807.

4. Gijsbers and Nicholson, "Experimental Pain Thresholds."

5. J. C. Ballantyne, "Gender, Pain, and the Brain," *Pain Clin Updates* 16, no. 3 (2008): 1–4.

6. Y. R. Smith et al., "Pronociceptive and Antinociceptive Effects of Estradiol Through Endogenous Opioid Neurotransmission in Women," *J Neurosci* 26, no. 21 (2006): 5777–5785.

7. A. Kaergaard et al., "Association Between Plasma Testosterone and Work-Related Neck and Shoulder Disorders Among Female Workers," *Scand J Work Environ Health* 26, no. 4 (2000): 292–298.

8. E. Keogh et al., "Comparing Acceptance-and Control-Based Coping In-structions on the Cold-Pressor Pain Experiences of Healthy Men and Women," *Eur J Pain* 9, no. 5 (2005): 591–598.

9. P. E. Bijur et al., "Response to Morphine in Male and Female Patients: Analgesia and Adverse Events," *Clin J Pain* 24, no. 3 (2008): 192–198.

10. F. Aubrun et al., "Sex-and Age-Related Differences in Morphine Require-ments for Postoperative Pain Relief," *Anesthesiology* 103, no. 1 (2005): 156–160.

11. R. W. Gear et al., "A Subanalgesic Dose of Morphine Eliminates Nal-buphine Anti-Analgesia in Postoperative Pain," *J Pain* 9, no. 4 (2008): 337–341; J. S. Mogil et al., "The Melanocortin-1 Receptor Gene Mediates Female-Specific Mechanisms of Analgesia in Mice and Humans," *Proc Natl Acad Sci USA* 100, no. 8 (2003): 4867–4872.

NOTES TO CHAPTER THREE

1. A. S. Gordon et al., "Characteristics of Women with Vulvar Pain Disor-ders: Responses to a Web-Based Survey," *J Sex Marital Ther* 29, Suppl. 1 (2003): 45–58.

2. "Doctors' Interpersonal Skills Valued More Than Their Training or Be-ing Up-to-Date," Harris Interactive, October 1, 2004, accessed December 28, 2009, www.harrisinteractive.com/news/allnewsbydate.asp?NewsID=850.

3. A. Nicolosi et al., "Sexual Behavior and Sexual Dysfunctions After Age 40: The Global Study of Sexual Attitudes and Behaviors," *Urology* 64, no. 5 (2004): 991–997.

4. S. Kingsberg, "Just Ask! Talking to Patients About Sexual Function," 2, no. 4 (2004): 199–203.

5. C. Marwick, "Survey Says Patients Expect Little Physician Help on Sex," *JAMA* 281, no. 23 (1999): 2173–2174.

NOTES TO CHAPTER FOUR

1. M. Ponte et al., "Effects of Vulvodynia on Quality of Life," *J Am Acad Dermatol* 60, no. 1 (2009): 70–76.

2. S. Sackett et al., "Psychosexual Aspects of Vulvar Vestibulitis," *J Reprod Med* 46, no. 6 (2001): 593–598.

3. Arnold et al., "Vulvodynia"; D. G. Tincello and A. C. Walker, "Intersti-tial Cystitis in the UK: Results of a Questionnaire Survey of Members of the Interstitial Cystitis Support Group," *Eur J Obstet Gynecol Reprod Biol* 118, no. 1 (2005): 91–95.

4. Arnold et al., "Vulvodynia."

5. K. B. Smith, C. F. Pukall, and S. C. Boyer, "Psychological and Relational Aspects of Dyspareunia," in *Female Sexual Pain Disorders: Evaluation and Management*, ed. A. Goldstein, C. F. Pukall, and I. Goldstein (New York: Wiley Blackwell, 2009), 208–212.

6. Sackett et al., "Psychosexual Aspects of Vulvar Vestibulitis"; B. D. Reed et al., "Sexual Activities and Attitudes of Women with Vulvar Dysesthesia," *Obstet Gynecol* 102, no. 2 (2003): 325–331; G. White and M. Jantos, "Sexual Behavior Changes with Vulvar Vestibulitis Syndrome," *J Reprod Med* 43, no. 9 (1998): 783–789; E. A. Gates and R. P. Galask, "Psychological and Sexual Functioning in Women with Vulvar Vestibulitis," *J Psychosom Obstet Gynaecol* 22, no. 4 (2001): 221–228.

7. White and Jantos, "Sexual Behavior Changes."

8. M. Desrosiers et al., "Psychosexual Characteristics of Vestibulodynia Couples: Partner Solicitousness and Hostility Are Associated with Pain," *J Sex Med* 5, no. 2 (2008): 418–427.

9. Desrosiers et al., "Psychosexual Characteristics of Vestibulodynia Couples."

10. Desrosiers et al., "Psychosexual Characteristics of Vestibulodynia Couples."

11. Desrosiers et al., "Psychosexual Characteristics of Vestibulodynia Couples."

12. I. Fernandez, C. Reid, and S. Dziurawiec, "Living with Endometriosis: The Perspective of Male Partners," *J Psychosom Res* 61, no. 4 (2006): 433–438; E. Nylanderlundqvist and J. Bergdahl, "Vulvar Vestibulitis: Evidence of Depression and State Anxiety in Patients and Partners," *Acta Derm Venereol* 83, no. 5 (2003): 369–373.

13. M. Meana et al., "Affect and Marital Adjustment in Women's Rating of Dyspareunic Pain," *Can J Psychiatry* 43, no. 4 (1998): 381–385.

NOTES TO CHAPTER FIVE

1. H. K. Haefner, "Report of the International Society for the Study of Vulvovaginal Disease Terminology and Classification of Vulvodynia," *J Low Genit Tract Dis* 11, no. 1 (2007): 48–49.

2. B. L. Harlow and E. G. Stewart, "A Population-Based Assessment of Chronic Unexplained Vulvar Pain: Have We Underestimated the Prevalence of Vulvodynia?" *J Am Med Women's Assoc* 58, no. 2 (2003): 82–88.

3. H. I. Glazer et al., "Electromyographic Comparisons of the Pelvic Floor in Women with Dysesthetic Vulvodynia and Asymptomatic Women," *J Reprod Med* 43, no. 11 (1998): 959–962.

4. H. I. Glazer, "Dysesthetic Vulvodynia: Long-Term Follow-Up After Treatment with Surface Electromyography-Assisted Pelvic Floor Muscle Rehabilitation," *J Reprod Med* 45, no. 10 (2000): 798–802.

5. D. G. Ferris et al., "Over-the-Counter Antifungal Drug Misuse Associated with Patient-Diagnosed Vulvovaginal Candidiasis," *Obstet Gynecol* 99, no. 3 (2002): 419–425.

6. G. Harris, B. Horowitz, and A. Borgida, "Evaluation of Gabapentin in the Treatment of Generalized Vulvodynia, Unprovoked," *J Reprod Med* 52, no. 2 (2007): 103–106.

7. J. Aranda and L. Edwards, *ISSVD World Congress.* Vol. 2007.

8. A. J. Rapkin, J. S. McDonald, and M. Morgan, "Multilevel Local Anesthetic Nerve Blockade for the Treatment of Vulvar Vestibulitis Syndrome," *Am J Obstet Gynecol* 198, no. 1 (2008): 41–45.

NOTES TO CHAPTER SIX

1. Harlow and Stewart, "A Population-Based Assessment."

2. P. Schweinhardt et al., "Increased Gray Matter Density in Young Women with Chronic Vulvar Pain," *Pain* 140, no. 3 (2008): 411–419.

3. C. F. Pukall et al., "Neural Correlates of Painful Genital Touch in Women with Vulvar Vestibulitis Syndrome," *Pain* 115, nos. 1–2 (2005): 118–127.

4. C. Bouchard et al., "Use of Oral Contraceptive Pills and Vulvar Vestibulitis: A Case-Control Study," *Am J Epidemiol* 156, no. 3 (2002): 254–261.

5. A. Greenstein et al., "Vulvar Vestibulitis Syndrome and Estrogen Dose of Oral Contraceptive Pills," *J Sex Med* 4, no. 6 (2007): 1679–1683.

6. C. Panzer et al., "Impact of Oral Contraceptives on Sex Hormone-Binding Globulin and Androgen Levels: A Retrospective Study in Women with Sexual Dysfunction," *J Sex Med* 3, no. 1 (2006): 104–113.

7. C. Goldfinger et al., "A Prospective Study of Pelvic Floor Physical Therapy: Pain and Psychosexual Outcomes in Provoked Vestibulodynia," *J Sex Med* 6, no. 7 (2009): 1955–1968.

8. C. Pukall et al., "Effectiveness of Hypnosis for the Treatment of Vulvar Vestibulitis Syndrome: A Preliminary Investigation," *Journal of Sexual Medicine* 4, no. 2 (2007): 417–425.

9. L. J. Burrows et al., "Umbilical Hypersensitivity in Women with Primary Vestibulodynia," *J Reprod Med* 53, no. 6 (2008): 413–416.

10. Burrows et al., "Umbilical Hypersensitivity."

11. C. F. Pukall et al., "The Vulvalgesiometer As a Device to Measure Genital Pressure-Pain Threshold," *Physiol Meas* 28, no. 12 (2007): 1543–1550.

12. C. F. Pukall, Y. M. Binik, and S. Khalife, "A New Instrument for Pain Assessment in Vulvar Vestibulitis Syndrome," *J Sex Marital Ther* 30, no. 2 (2004): 69–78.

13. Burrows et al., "Umbilical Hypersensitivity."

14. O. Babula et al., "Association Between Primary Vulvar Vestibulitis Syndrome, Defective Induction of Tumor Necrosis Factor-Alpha, and Carriage of the Mannose-Binding Lectin Codon 54 Gene Polymorphism," *Am J Obstet Gynecol* 198, no. 1 (2008): 101–104.

15. J. Bornstein, N. Goldschmid, and E. Sabo, "Hyperinnervation and Mast Cell Activation May Be Used As Histopathologic Diagnostic Criteria for Vulvar Vestibulitis," *Gynecol Obstet Invest* 58, no. 3 (2004): 171–178.

16. A. T. Goldstein et al., "Interferon Alpha Therapy for Vulvar Vestibulitis Syndrome: A Large Retrospective Trial" (poster presented at the International Society for the Study of Women's Sexual Health, Vancouver, British Columbia, October 2002).

17. D. A. Zolnoun, K. E. Hartmann, and J. F. Steege, "Overnight 5% Lidocaine Ointment for Treatment of Vulvar Vestibulitis," *Obstet Gynecol* 102, no. 1 (2003): 84–87.

18. L. A. Boardman et al., "Topical Gabapentin in the Treatment of Localized and Generalized Vulvodynia," *Obstet Gynecol* 112, no. 3 (2008): 579–585.

19. A. T. Goldstein et al., "Surgical Treatment of Vulvar Vestibulitis Syndrome: Outcome Assessment Derived from a Postoperative Questionnaire," *J Sex Med* 3, no. 5 (2006): 923–931.

20. M. S. Baggish, E. H. Sze, and R. Johnson, "Urinary Oxalate Excretion and Its Role in Vulvar Pain Syndrome," *Am J Obstet Gynecol* 177, no. 3 (1997): 507–511.

21. A. V. Sarma et al., "Epidemiology of Vulvar Vestibulitis Syndrome: An Exploratory Case-Control Study," *Sex Transm Infect* 75, no. 5 (1999): 320–326.

22. B. L. Harlow et al., "Influence of Dietary Oxalates on the Risk of Adult-Onset Vulvodynia," *J Reprod Med* 53, no. 3 (2008): 171–178.

NOTES TO CHAPTER SEVEN

1. "CDC Study Finds US Herpes Rates Remain High," Centers for Disease Control and Prevention, March 9, 2010, accessed March 10, 2010, www.cdc.gov/nchhstp/Newsroom/hsv2pressrelease.html.

2. J. F. Steege and A. L. Stout, "Resolution of Chronic Pelvic Pain After Laparoscopic Lysis of Adhesions," *Am J Obstet Gynecol* 165, no. 2 (1991): 278–281; discussion 281–273.

3. M. Sutton et al., "The Prevalence of Trichomonas Vaginalis Infection Among Reproductive-Age Women in the United States, 2001–2004," *Clin Infect Dis* 45, no. 10 (2007): 1319–1326.

4. Z. F. Zhang and C. B. Begg, "Is Trichomonas Vaginalis a Cause of Cervical Neoplasia? Results from a Combined Analysis of 24 Studies," *Int J Epidemiol*

23, no. 4 (1994): 682–690; A. M. El-Shazly et al., "A Study on Trichomoniasis Vaginalis and Female Infertility," *J Egypt Soc Parasitol* 31, no. 2 (2001): 545–553.

5. M. Laga et al., "Non-Ulcerative Sexually Transmitted Diseases As Risk Factors for HIV-1 Transmission in Women: Results from a Cohort Study," *AIDS* 7, no. 1 (1993): 95–102.

6. "Pudendal Neuralgia," Cure Together, accessed March 18, 2010, www.curetogether.com/pudendal-neuralgia/symptoms.

7. L. D. Arnold et al., "Assessment of Vulvodynia Symptoms in a Sample of US Women: A Prevalence Survey with a Nested Case Control Study," *Am J Obstet Gynecol* 196, no. 2 (2007): 121–126.

8. J. D. Sobel, "Vulvovaginal Candidosis," *Lancet* 369, no. 9577 (2007): 1961–1971.

9. M. Pirotta et al., "Effect of Lactobacillus in Preventing Post-Antibiotic Vulvovaginal Candidiasis: A Randomised Controlled Trial," *BMJ* 329, no. 7465 (2004): 548.

10. L. A. Sadownik, "Clinical Profile of Vulvodynia Patients: A Prospective Study of 300 Patients," *J Reprod Med* 45, no. 8 (2000): 679–684.

11. E. Rylander et al., "Vulvovaginal Candida in a Young Sexually Active Population: Prevalence and Association with Oro-Genital Sex and Frequent Pain at Intercourse," *Sex Transm Infect* 80, no. 1 (2004): 54–57.

12. J. D. Sobel, "Candidal Vulvovaginitis," *Clin Obstet Gynecol* 36, no. 1 (1993): 153–165.

13. Sobel, "Vulvovaginal Candidosis."

14. N. K. Lowe, J. L. Neal, and N. A. Ryan-Wenger, "Accuracy of the Clinical Diagnosis of Vaginitis Compared with a DNA Probe Laboratory Standard," *Obstet Gynecol* 113, no. 1 (2009): 89–95.

15. A. Spinillo et al., "Effect of Antibiotic Use on the Prevalence of Symptomatic Vulvovaginal Candidiasis," *Am J Obstet Gynecol* 180, no. 1, pt. 1 (1999): 14–17.

16. J. D. Sobel, "What's New in Bacterial Vaginosis and Trichomoniasis?" *Infect Dis Clin North Am* 19, no. 2 (2005): 387–406; M. R. Joesoef and G. Schmid, "Bacterial Vaginosis," *Clin Evid* 13 (2005): 1968–1978.

NOTES TO CHAPTER EIGHT

1. "Pudendal Neuralgia," Cure Together, accessed March 18, 2010, www.curetogether.com/pudendal-neuralgia/symptoms.

2. A. Goldstein and C. F. Pukall, *Female Sexual Pain Disorders: Evaluation and Management* (New York: Wiley-Blackwell, 2009).

NOTES TO CHAPTER NINE

1. T. G. Stovall, F. W. Ling, and D. A. Crawford, "Hysterectomy for Chronic Pelvic Pain of Presumed Uterine Etiology," *Obstet Gynecol* 75, no. 4 (1990): 676–679.

2. K. T. Zondervan et al., "Patterns of Diagnosis and Referral in Women Consulting for Chronic Pelvic Pain in UK Primary Care," *Br J Obstet Gynaecol* 106, no. 11 (1999): 1156–1161.

3. M. K. Chung and B. Jarnagin, "Early Identification of Interstitial Cystitis May Avoid Unnecessary Hysterectomy," *JSLS* 13, no. 3 (2009): 350–357.

4. N. M. Cinman, C. Huckabay, and R. M. Moldwin, "Interstitial Cystitis and Dyspareunia," in *Female Sexual Pain Disorders: Evaluation and Management*, ed. A. Goldstein, C. F. Pukall, and I. Goldstein (New York: Wiley-Blackwell, 2009), 88–94.

5. Cinman, Huckabay, and Moldwin, "Interstitial Cystitis and Dyspareunia."

6. J. Adams et al., "Uterine Size and Endometrial Thickness and the Significance of Cystic Ovaries in Women with Pelvic Pain Due to Congestion," *Br J Obstet Gynaecol* 97, no. 7 (1990): 583–587.

7. E. Kuligowska, L. Deeds III, and K. Lu III, "Pelvic Pain: Overlooked and Underdiagnosed Gynecologic Conditions," *Radiographics* 25, no. 1 (2005): 3–20.

8. Kuligowska, Deeds, and Lu, "Pelvic Pain."

9. S. Ferrero et al., "Deep Dyspareunia and Sex Life After Laparoscopic Excision of Endometriosis," *Hum Reprod* 22, no. 4 (2007): 1142–1148.

10. J. Droz and F. M. Howard, "Endometriosis," in *Female Sexual Pain Disorders: Evaluation and Management*, ed. A. Goldstein, C. F. Pukall, and I. Goldstein (New York: Wiley-Blackwell, 2009), 124–130.

11. R. L. Barbieri, S. Evans, and R. W. Kistner, "Danazol in the Treatment of Endometriosis: Analysis of 100 Cases with a 4-Year Follow-Up," *Fertil Steril* 37, no. 6 (1982): 737–746.

12. M. D. Hornstein et al., "Leuprolide Acetate Depot and Hormonal Add-Back in Endometriosis: A 12-Month Study," *Obstet Gynecol* 91, no. 1 (1998): 16–24.

13. P. Vercellini et al., "A Gonadotropin-Releasing Hormone Agonist Versus a Low-Dose Oral Contraceptive for Pelvic Pain Associated with Endometriosis," *Fertil Steril* 60, no. 1 (1993): 75–79.

14. F. M. Howard, "Laparoscopic Evaluation and Treatment of Women with Chronic Pelvic Pain," *J Am Assoc Gynecol Laparosc* 1, no. 4, pt. 1 (1994): 325–331.

15. J. Abbott et al., "Laparoscopic Excision of Endometriosis: A Randomized, Placebo-Controlled Trial," *Fertil Steril* 82, no. 4 (2004): 878–884.

16. F. Zullo et al., "Effectiveness of Presacral Neurectomy in Women with Severe Dysmenorrhea Caused by Endometriosis Who Were Treated with Laparoscopic Conservative Surgery: A 1-Year Prospective Randomized Double-Blind Controlled Trial," *Am J Obstet Gynecol* 189, no. 1 (2003): 5–10.

17. A. B. Namnoum et al., "Incidence of Symptom Recurrence After Hysterectomy for Endometriosis," *Fertil Steril* 64, no. 5 (1995): 898–902.

18. G. F. Longstreth et al., "Functional Bowel Disorders," in *Rome III: The Functional Gastrointestinal Disorders*, ed. D. A. Drossman et al. (McLean, VA: Degnon Associates, Inc., 2006), 487–555; F. Cremonini and N. J. Talley, "Irritable Bowel Syndrome: Epidemiology, Natural History, Health Care Seeking and Emerging Risk Factors," *Gastroenterol Clin N Amer* 34 (2005): 189–204; A. P. Hungin et al., "The Prevalence, Patterns and Impact of Irritable Bowel Syndrome: An International Survey of 40,000 Subjects," *Aliment Pharmacol Ther* 17 (2003): 643–650; D. A. Drossman et al., "U.S. Householder Survey of Functional GI Disorders: Prevalence, Sociodemography and Health Impact," *Dig Dis Sci* 38 (1993): 1569–1580.

19. G. Longstreth, D. B. Preskill, and L. Youkeles. "Irritable Bowel Syndrome in Women Having Diagnostic Laparoscopy or Hysterectomy: Relation to Gynecologic Features and Outcome," *Dig Dis Sci* 35 (1990): 1285–1290.

20. D. A. Drossman, "The Functional Gastrointestinal Disorders and the Rome III Process," in *Rome III: The Functional Gastrointestinal Disorders*, ed. D. A. Drossman et al., 2nd ed. (McLean, VA: Degnon Associates, Inc., 2006), 1–29; A. R. Hobson and Q. Aziz, "Brain Imaging and Functional Gastrointestinal Disorders: Has It Helped Our Understanding?" *Gut* 53 (2004): 1198–1206; E. A. Mayer et al., "V. Stress and Irritable Bowel Syndrome," *Am J Physiol Gastrointest Liver Physiol* 280 (2001): G519–G524; J. D. Wood et al., "Fundamentals of Neurogastroenterology: Basic Science," in *Rome III: The Functional Gastrointestinal Disorders*, ed. D. A. Drossman et al., 3rd ed. (McLean, VA: Degnon Associates, Inc., 2006).

21. A. D. Sperber et al., "Development of Abdominal Pain and IBS Following Gynecological Surgery: A Prospective, Controlled Study," *Gastroenterology* 134 (2008): 75–84.

22. C. F. Pukall et al., "Neural Correlates of Painful Genital Touch in Women with Vulvar Vestibulitis Syndrome," *Pain* 115 (2005): 118–127; C. F. Pukall et al., "Vestibular Tactile and Pain Thresholds in Women with Vulvar Vestibulitis Syndrome," *Pain* 96 (2002): 163–175.

23. Longstreth, Preskill, and Youkeles. "Irritable Bowel Syndrome in Women"; P. J. Whorwell et al., "Non-Colonic Features of Irritable Bowel Syndrome," *Gut* 27 (1986): 37–40; A. Prior et al., "Irritable Bowel Syndrome in the Gynecological Clinic: Survey of 798 New Referrals," *Dig Dis Sci* 34 (1989): 1820–1824; K. T. Zondervan et al., "Chronic Pelvic Pain in the Community: Symptoms, Investigations, and Diagnoses," *Am J Obstet Gynecol* 184 (2001): 1149–1155.

24. E. A. Walker et al., "The Prevalence of Chronic Pelvic Pain and Irritable Bowel Syndrome in Two University Clinics," *J Psychosom Obstet Gynaecol* 12 suppl. (1991): 65–75; G. F. Longstreth, "Irritable Bowel Syndrome and Chronic Pelvic Pain," *Obstet Gynecol Survey* 49 (1994): 505–507.

25. Whorwell et al., "Non-Colonic Features of Irritable Bowel Syndrome"; Walker et al., "The Prevalence of Chronic Pelvic Pain"; R. Fass et al., "Sexual Dysfunction in Patients with Irritable Bowel Syndrome and Non-Ulcer Dyspepsia," *Digestion* 59 (1998): 79–85; R. H. Corney and R. Stanton, "Physical Symptom Severity, Psychological and Social Dysfunction in a Series of Outpatients with Irritable Bowel Syndrome," *J Psychosom Res* 34 (1990): 483–491.

26. D. M. Owens, D. K. Nelson, and N. J. Talley, "The Irritable Bowel Syndrome: Long-Term Prognosis and the Physician-Patient Interaction," *Ann Intern Med* 122, no. 2 (1995): 107–112.

27. G. F. Longstreth et al., "Functional Bowel Disorders," *Gastroenterology* 130, no. 5 (2006): 1480–1491.

28. I. L. Zijdenbos et al., "Psychological Treatments for the Management of Irritable Bowel Syndrome," *Cochrane Database Syst Rev* 1 (2009): CD006442; D. A. Drossman and W. G. Thompson, "The Irritable Bowel Syndrome: Review and a Graduated Multicomponent Treatment Approach," *Ann Intern Med* 116, no. 12, pt. 1 (1992): 1009–1016.

29. A. C. Ford et al., "Efficacy of Antidepressants and Psychological Therapies in Irritable Bowel Syndrome: Systematic Review and Meta-Analysis," *Gut* 58, no. 3 (2009): 367–378.

NOTES TO CHAPTER TEN

1. A. T. Goldstein et al., "Prevalence of Vulvar Lichen Sclerosus in a General Gynecology Practice," *J Reprod Med* 50, no. 7 (2005): 477–480.

2. A. T. Goldstein et al., "Topical Calcineurin Inhibitors for the Treatment of Vulvar Dermatoses," *Eur J Obstet Gynecol Reprod Biol* 146, no. 1 (2009): 22–29.

3. A. T. Goldstein et al., "A Double Blind, Parallel-Group Trial of Topical Pimecrolimus Cream Versus Clobetasol Cream for the Treatment of Vulvar Lichen Sclerosus," *J Lower Genital Tract Dis* (October 2009): S9.

4. A. T. Goldstein and L. J. Burrows. "Surgical Treatment of Clitoral Phimosis Caused by Lichen Sclerosus," *Am J Obstet Gynecol* 196, no. 2 (2007): 126.e1–4; I. Goldstein, "Dorsal Slit Surgery for Clitoral Phimosis," *J Sex Med* 5, no. 11 (2008): 2485–2488.

5. L. J. Burrows et al., "Vulvar Dermatoses As a Cause of Dsypareunia," in *Female Sexual Pain Disorders: Evaluation and Management*, ed. A. Goldstein, C. F. Pukall, and I. Goldstein (New York: Wiley-Blackwell, 2009), 49–56.

6. Burrows et al., "Vulvar Dermatoses As a Cause of Dsypareunia."

7. J. M. Rhode, A. S. Kueck, and H. K. Haefner, "Hidradenitis Suppurativa," in *Female Sexual Pain Disorders: Evaluation and Management*, ed. A. Goldstein, C. F. Pukall, and I. Goldstein (New York: Wiley-Blackwell, 2009), 57–65.

8. Rhode, Kueck, and Haefner, "Hidradenitis Suppurativa."

9. P. Haslund, R. A. Lee, and G. B. Jemec, "Treatment of Hidradenitis Suppurativa with Tumour Necrosis Factor-Alpha Inhibitors," *Acta Derm Venereol* 89, no. 6 (2009): 595–600; G. B. Jemec, "Medical Treatment of Hidradenitis Suppurativa," *Expert Opin Pharmacother* 5, no. 8 (2004): 1767–1770.

NOTES TO CHAPTER ELEVEN

1. "Sexual Violence," Centers for Disease Control and Prevention, spring 2008, accessed September 28, 2010, www.cdc.gov/ViolencePrevention/sexual violence.

2. P. Latthe et al., "Factors Predisposing Women to Chronic Pelvic Pain: Systematic Review," *BMJ* 332 (2006): 749–755.

3. F. E. Springs and W. N. Friedrich, "Health Risk Behaviors and Medical Sequelae of Childhood Sexual Abuse," *Mayo Clin Proc* 67, no. 6 (1992): 527–532.

4. B. D. Reed et al., "Psychosocial and Sexual Functioning in Women with Vulvodynia and Chronic Pelvic Pain: A Comparative Evaluation," *J Reprod Med* 45, no. 8 (2000): 624–632; R. Bodden-Heidrich et al., "Chronic Pelvic Pain Syndrome (CPPS) and Chronic Vulvar Pain Syndrome (CVPS): Evaluation of Psychosomatic Aspects," *J Psychosom Obstet Gynaecol* 20, no. 3 (1999): 145–151; A. Lampe et al., "Chronic Pelvic Pain and Previous Sexual Abuse," *Obstet Gynecol* 96, no. 6 (2000): 929–933; A. Matheis et al., "Irritable Bowel Syndrome and Chronic Pelvic Pain: A Singular or Two Different Clinical Syndromes?" *World J Gastroenterol* 13, no. 25 (2007): 3446–3455; B. W. Fenton, C. Durner, and J. Fanning, "Frequency and Distribution of Multiple Diagnoses in Chronic Pelvic Pain Related to Previous Abuse or Drug-Seeking Behavior," *Gynecol Obstet Invest* 65, no. 4 (2008): 247–251; K. M. Peters et al., "Fact or Fiction—Is Abuse Prevalent in Patients with Interstitial Cystitis? Results from a Community Survey and Clinic Population," *J Urol* 178, no. 3, pt. 1 (2007): 891–895; discussion 895; N. J. Talley et al., "Gastrointestinal Tract Symptoms and Self-Reported Abuse: A Population-Based Study," *Gastroenterology* 107, no. 4 (1994): 1040–1049.

5. Matheis et al., "Irritable Bowel Syndrome and Chronic Pelvic Pain"; Peters et al., "Fact or Fiction."

6. D. A. Drossman et al., "Sexual and Physical Abuse in Women with Functional or Organic Gastrointestinal Disorders," *Ann Intern Med* 113 (1990): 828–833; E. A. Walker et al., "Histories of Sexual Victimization in Patients with Irritable Bowel Syndrome or Inflammatory Bowel Disease," *Am J Psychiatry* 150

(1993): 1502–1506; D. A. Drossman et al., "Sexual and Physical Abuse and Gastrointestinal Illness: Review and Recommendations," *Ann Intern Med* 123, no. 10 (1995): 782–794; D. A. Drossman et al., "Health Status by Gastrointestinal Diagnosis and Abuse History," *Gastroenterology* 110 (1996): 999–1007.

7. B. D. Reed, "Dyspaurenia and Sexual/Physical Abuse," in *Female Sexual Pain Disorders: Evaluation and Management*, ed. A. Goldstein, C. F. Pukall, and I. Goldstein (New York: Wiley-Blackwell, 2009), 213–217.

8. Reed, "Dyspaurenia and Sexual/Physical Abuse."

9. A. Lampe et al., "Chronic Pain Syndromes and Their Relation to Childhood Abuse and Stressful Life Events," *J Psychosom Res* 54, no. 4 (2003): 361–367.

10. B. W. Fenton, "Limbic Associated Pelvic Pain: A Hypothesis to Explain the Diagnostic Relationships and Features of Patients with Chronic Pelvic Pain," *Med Hypotheses* 69, no. 2 (2007): 282–286.

11. D. A. Drossman et al., "Alterations of Brain Activity Associated with Resolution of Emotional Distress and Pain in a Case of Severe Irritable Bowel Syndrome," *Gastroenterology* 124 (2003): 754–761.

12. Y. Ringel et al., "Effect of Abuse History on Pain Reports and Brain Responses to Aversive Visceral Stimulation: An fMRI Study," *Gastroenterology* 134, no. 2 (2008): 396–404.

NOTES TO CHAPTER TWELVE

1. K. Klein et al., "Does the Mode of Delivery Influence Sexual Function After Childbirth?" *J Women's Health* (Larchmt) 18, no. 8 (2009): 1227–1231; C. MacNeil, M. F. Davies, and J. T. Repke, "Postpartum Dyspareunia," in *Female Sexual Pain Disorders: Evaluation and Management*, ed. A. Goldstein, C. F. Pukall, and I. Goldstein (New York: Wiley-Blackwell, 2009), 224–228.

2. MacNeil, Davies, and Repke, "Postpartum Dyspareunia."

3. Klein et al., "Does the Mode of Delivery Influence Sexual Function After Childbirth?"; V. Andrews et al., "Evaluation of Postpartum Perineal Pain and Dyspareunia—a Prospective Study," *Eur J Obstet Gynecol Reprod Biol* 137, no. 2 (2008): 152–156.

4. L. B. Signorello et al., "Postpartum Sexual Functioning and Its Relationship to Perineal Trauma: A Retrospective Cohort Study of Primiparous Women," *Am J Obstet Gynecol* 184, no. 5 (2001): 881–888; discussion 888–890; H. Ejegard, E. L. Ryding, and B. Sjogren, "Sexuality After Delivery with Episiotomy: A Long-Term Follow-Up," *Gynecol Obstet Invest* 66, no. 1 (2008): 1–7; P. G. Larsson et al., "Advantage or Disadvantage of Episiotomy Compared with Spontaneous Perineal Laceration," *Gynecol Obstet Invest* 31, no. 4 (1991): 213–216.

5. G. Carroli and L. Mignini, "Episiotomy for Vaginal Birth," *Cochrane Database Syst Rev* 1 (2009): CD000081.

6. Klein et al., "Does the Mode of Delivery Influence Sexual Function After Childbirth?"

7. A. Connolly, J. Thorp, and L. Pahel, "Effects of Pregnancy and Childbirth on Postpartum Sexual Function: A Longitudinal Prospective Study," *Int Urogynecol J Pelvic Floor Dysfunct* 16, no. 4 (2005): 263–267; G. Barrett et al., "Women's Sexual Health After Childbirth," *BJOG* 107, no. 2 (2000): 186–195.

8. C. Fleten et al., "Exercise During Pregnancy, Maternal Prepregnancy Body Mass Index, and Birth Weight," *Obstet Gynecol* 115, no. 2, pt. 1 (2010): 331–337.

9. M. M. Beckmann and A. J. Garrett, "Antenatal Perineal Massage for Reducing Perineal Trauma," *Cochrane Database Syst Rev* 1 (2006): CD005123.

10. A. Grant et al., "The Ipswich Childbirth Study: One Year Follow-Up of Alternative Methods Used in Perineal Repair," *BJOG* 108, no. 1 (2001): 34–40.

11. G. Davis and J. Brooks, "Pelvic Organ Prolapse and Sexual Pain," in *Female Sexual Pain Disorders: Evaluation and Management*, ed. A. Goldstein, C. F. Pukall, and I. Goldstein (New York: Wiley-Blackwell, 2009), 143–149.

12. C. Maher et al., "Surgical Management of Pelvic Organ Prolapse in Women," *Cochrane Database Syst Rev* 4 (2010): CD004014.

13. L. Pastore, A. Owens, and C. Raymond, "Postpartum Sexuality Concerns Among First-Time Parents from One U.S. Academic Hospital," *J Sex Med* 4, no. 1 (2007): 115–123.

14. Zolnoun, Hartmann, and Steege, "Overnight 5% Lidocaine Ointment."

NOTES TO CHAPTER THIRTEEN

1. M. Redelman, "A General Look at Female Orgasm and Anorgasmia," *Sex Health* 3, no. 3 (2006): 143–153.

2. D. Hartmann and C. A. Nelson, "The Perceived Effectiveness of Physical Therapy Treatment on Women Complaining of Chronic Vulvar Pain and Diagnosed with Either Vulvar Vestibulitis Syndrome or Dysetheic Vulvodynia," *J Sect Women's Health APTA* 25 (2001): 13–18.

3. Goldfinger et al., "A Prospective Study of Pelvic Floor Physical Therapy"; E. Gentilcore-Saulnier et al., "Pelvic Floor Muscle Assessment Outcomes in Women with and without Provoked Vestibulodynia and the Impact of a Physical Therapy Program," *J Sex Med* 7 (2010): 1003–1022.

4. T. Rosenbaum, "Physical Therapy Evaluation of Dyspareunia," in *Female Sexual Pain Disorders: Evaluation and Management*, ed. A. Goldstein, C. F. Pukall, and I. Goldstein (New York: Wiley-Blackwell, 2009), 27–31.

5. Glazer et al., "Electromyographic Comparisons of the Pelvic Floor."

6. D. Hartmann, M. J. Strauhal, and C. A. Nelson, "Treatment of Women in the United States with Localized, Provoked Vulvodynia: Practice Survey of Women's Health Physical Therapists," *J Reprod Med* 52, no. 1 (2007): 48–52.

NOTES TO CHAPTER FOURTEEN

1. S. Bergeron et al., "A Randomized Comparison of Group Cognitive-Behavioral Therapy, Surface Electromyographic Biofeedback, and Vestibulectomy in the Treatment of Dyspareunia Resulting from Vulvar Vestibulitis," *Pain* 91, no. 3 (2001): 297–306.

2. S. Bergeron et al., "Surgical and Behavioral Treatments for Vestibulodynia: Two-and-One-Half Year Follow-Up and Predictors of Outcome," *Obstet Gynecol* 111, no. 1 (2008): 159–166.

3. S. Bergeron, T. Landry, and B. Leclerc, "Cognitive-Behavioral, Physical Therapy, and Alternative Treatments for Dyspareunia," in *Female Sexual Pain Disorders: Evaluation and Management*, ed. A. Goldstein, C. F. Pukall, and I. Goldstein (New York: Wiley-Blackwell, 2009), 150–155.

4. S. Bergeron, Y. M. Binik, and J. Larouche, *Cognitive Behavioral Pain and Sex Therapy Treatment Manual* (Montreal: McGill University Press, 2001).

NOTES TO CHAPTER SIXTEEN

1. A. Schneidewind-Skibbe et al., "The Frequency of Sexual Intercourse Reported by Women: A Review of Community-Based Studies and Factors Limiting Their Conclusions," *J Sex Med* 5, no. 2 (2008): 301–335.

2. S. A. Sanders and J. M. Reinisch, "Would You Say You 'Had Sex' if? . . ." *JAMA* 281, no. 3 (1999): 275–277.

3. D. A. Donnelly, "Sexually Inactive Marriages," *J Sex Res* 30, no. 2 (1993): 171–179.

4. R. J. Levin, "The Physiology and Pathophysiology of the Female Orgasm," in *Women's Sexual Function and Dysfunction: Study, Diagnosis and Treatment*, ed. I. Goldstein et al. (New York: Taylor & Francis, 2006).

5. A. Bartels and S. Zeki, "The Neural Basis of Romantic Love," *Neuroreport* 11, no. 17 (2000): 3829–3834.

6. E. R. R. Hatfield, "Love and Passion," in *Women's Sexual Function and Dysfunction: Study, Diagnosis and Treatment*, ed. I. Goldstein et al. (New York: Taylor & Francis, 2006).

7. P. Kleinplatz, "Aging—the Secret to Good Sex," *Can J Hum Sexuality* 18, nos. 1–2 (2009).

8. Hatfield, "Love and Passion."

9. R. Basson, "Recent Advances in Women's Sexual Function and Dysfunction," *Menopause* 11, no. 6, pt. 2 (2004): 714–725.

NOTES TO CHAPTER SEVENTEEN

1. A. T. Goldstein, "Moving Beyond the Diagnosis of Vestibulodynia," *J Sex Med* 6, no. 12 (2009): 3227–3229.

2. L. A. Boardman et al., "Topical Gabapentin in the Treatment of Localized and Generalized Vulvodynia," *Obstet Gynecol* 112, no. 3 (2008): 579–585.

3. A. Truini et al., "Laser-Evoked Potentials in Post-Herpetic Neuralgia," *Clin Neurophysiol* 114, no. 4 (2003): 702–709.

4. A. Bradford and C. Meston, "Correlates of Placebo Response in the Treatment of Sexual Dysfunction in Women: A Preliminary Report," *J Sex Med* 4, no. 5 (2007): 1345–1351.

5. M. Moyal-Barracco and P. J. Lynch, "2003 ISSVD Terminology and Classification of Vulvodynia: A Historical Perspective," *J Reprod Med* 49, no. 10 (2004): 772–777.

6. D. C. Foster, "The Future of Vulvodynia Research," in *Female Sexual Pain Disorders: Evaluation and Management*, ed. A. Goldstein, C. F. Pukall, and I. Goldstein (New York: Wiley-Blackwell, 2009), 255–260.

7. G. Lamvu and L. Boardman, "The National Provider-Based Vulvodynia Outcomes Registry," 2010.

8. Foster, "The Future of Vulvodynia Research."

9. Truini et al., "Laser-Evoked Potentials in Post-Herpetic Neuralgia."

10. D. C. Foster et al., "Enhanced Synthesis of Proinflammatory Cytokines by Vulvar Vestibular Fibroblasts: Implications for Vulvar Vestibulitis," *Am J Obstet Gynecol* 196, no. 4 (2007): 341–348.

11. D. Alonso et al., "Drugs from the Sea: Conotoxins As Drug Leads for Neuropathic Pain and Other Neurological Conditions," *Mini Rev Med Chem* 3, no. 7 (2003): 785–787; U. Klotz, "Ziconotide—a Novel Neuron-Specific Calcium Channel Blocker for the Intrathecal Treatment of Severe Chronic Pain—a Short Review," *Int J Clin Pharmacol Ther* 44, no. 10 (2006): 478–483.

12. M. M. Ibrahim et al., "CB2 Cannabinoid Receptor Mediation of Antinociception," *Pain* 122, nos. 1–2 (2006): 36–42.

13. T. Rohl and J. Kurreck, "RNA Interference in Pain Research," *J Neurochem* 99, no. 2 (2006): 371–380.

14. R. C. deCharms et al., "Control over Brain Activation and Pain Learned by Using Real-Time Functional MRI," *Proc Natl Acad Sci USA* 102, no. 51 (2005): 18626–18631.

⊘ Index

Doctor(s) *(continued)*
  appointment, preparation for, 38–40
  choice of, 34–38
  and diagnosis, 34, 35–37
  and doctor-patient confidentiality, 36
  and sexual pain, 6, 7
  and sexual pain as psychological
    problem, 34, 35–36
  and sexuality, women's, 6–7
  and treatment, questions to ask
    about, 47–48
  and vulvodynia, diagnosis of, 66–67
  See also Health-care professionals
Doxycycline, 105
Duloxetine (Cymbalta), 74, 92,
  125, 134
Dyspareunia
  causes of, 99–100
  and health-care professionals,
    experience with, 37
  research on, 215–221
  See also Pain; Sexual pain
Dyspareunia, 14

Education, 187–188
Effexor (venlafaxine), 74, 92, 221
Elavil (amitriptyline), 73, 92, 134,
  145, 157
Electrical stimulation, 182
Electromyelogram, 47
Electromyography, 89, 123
Elidel (pimecrolimus), 152–153, 156
Elmiron (pentosanpolysulfate), 134
Enbrel (etanercept), 158
Endometriosis, 15, 24, 136–141
  causes of, 137–138
  diagnosis of, 138–139
  treatment of, 139–141
Endometriotic implants, 137
Entrapment injury, 120–121
Epidemiological research, 217–218
Epidurals, 75
Episiotomy, 10
  and postpartum dyspareunia, 166,
    167, 168
Erosive lichen planus, 15

Escitalopram (Lexapro), 74
Estrogen, 96, 111, 115, 153, 167,
  171–172
  and desquamative inflammatory
    vaginitis, 114–116
  and postpartum dyspareunia,
    171–172
  and provoked vestibulodynia,
    98, 99
  See Reproductive hormones
Etanercept (Enbrel), 158
Exercise, 168, 178, 179–180, 181–182
Eye Movement Desensitization and
  Reprocessing, 162–163

Fallopian tubes, 12
Famiciclovir (Famvir), 103
Famvir (famiciclovir), 103
Female Sexual Function Index, 43
Fetal development, abnormal, 16–18
Fibromyalgia, 70
Finasteride (Proscar), 158
Flagyl (MetroGel; metronidazole), 105,
  106, 114, 115
Fluconazole (Diflucan), 109, 112
Fluoroquinolones, 105
Fluoxetine (Prozac), 74
Focused breathing, 28
Foods, 134

Gabapentin (Neurontin), 75, 92,
  125, 134, 216
Gardnerella, 96, 113
Gastrointestinal conditions, 16
Gender
  and pain, differences in, 28–31
  and pain medication, 31–32
  See also Men; Partners
Generalized vulvodynia (GVD),
  65–68, 69–70
  advice from women with, 77
  causes of, 15, 70
  diagnosis of, 71
  treatment of, 71–77
  See also Vulvodynia
Genetics, 30, 112, 113